Taking Care After 50

Medical Reviewers

Kathy S. Brenneman, MD, MPH
Director of Geriatric Medicine, Providence Hospital, Washington, DC

Todd A. Horwitz, MD, MBA
Vice President, Medical Management, Sierra Military Health Services, Baltimore, MD

Ken Maffet, MD, CPE, MACP
Chief Medical Officer, VHA Rocky Mountain Network, Glendale, CO

E. J. Smith, MD

Robert G. Harmon, MD, MPH, FACPM
Vice President and National Medical Director, Optum®

Phyllis DeCarlo Cross, MD, MPH
Medical Consultant, Optum

Bonnie J. Morcomb, RN, MS
Vice President, Operations, Optum

Marcie Parker, PhD, CFLE
Senior Qualitative Researcher, Optum

Editor
Susan Perry

Product Manager
Renee L. Pietrzak

Creative Director
Nancy Larson-Knott

Publications Manager
Linda Acorn

Taking Care After 50
A SELF-CARE GUIDE FOR SENIORS

by Harvey Jay Cohen, MD

Professor of Medicine and Director of the Center for the Study of Aging and Human Development at Duke University

THREE RIVERS PRESS • NEW YORK

Taking Care After 50 *is an excellent resource to help you develop a great working relationship with your health care provider. Understanding health concerns can help you ask the right questions and feel confident about making health care choices. While* **Taking Care After 50** *provides valuable information, you should not rely on it to replace necessary medical consultations to meet your individual health care needs.*

Cover design by Random House
Inside page design by Young Design

Library of Congress Cataloging-in-Publication Data
    Cohen, Harvey Jay.
        Taking care after 50 : a self-care guide for seniors / by Harvey Jay Cohen— 1st ed.
            p. cm.
        Includes bibliographical references and index.
        1. Aged—Health and hygiene. 2. Self-care, Health. I. Title: Taking care after fifty. II. Title.
RA777.6.C64 2000
613'.0438--dc21   00-060731
Three Rivers Press ISBN 0-8129-3174-2
United HealthCare Services ISBN 0-8129-9045-5
10 9
First Edition

Contents

Contents

A NOTE FROM THE AUTHOR

Each year, more and more people turn 50 and enter their second half century. Although each passing birthday leaves us more vulnerable to disease- and age-related changes, most older Americans live independently, actively, and well.

There are many things you can do to maximize your potential for a healthy, productive, and enjoyable life well into old age. Obtaining good medical and health care is one, of course. But you can also take many preventive and self-care actions to ensure good health after age 50.

That's what this book is all about. It provides you with easy-to-use information on ways to promote a healthy lifestyle. It also teaches you how to understand and handle medical problems that may arise as you grow older.

We have used the term "nurse information service" throughout the book for those people who have telephone access to a nurse as part of their health plan or through their employer. If you do not have a nurse information service, then simply call your doctor's office instead.

You'll also note that we have put in **boldface** illnesses and conditions that have separate entries in the book. We hope this cross-referencing will help speed your search for more information on these topics.

The first section, "Prescription for Health," lists eight habits for healthful aging—good, detailed ideas for how you can begin to make more healthful choices in your life.

Starting on page 55, you'll find a section called "Major Health Concerns." It describes the symptoms, causes, treatments, and much more for the most prevalent chronic, or long-term, diseases that affect older people. You'll also find tips for how to prevent these illnesses and, when appropriate, recommendations for at-home care. Because a chronic ailment can be life-altering, we also offer suggestions on how you can learn to adjust to living with these conditions, emotionally as well as physically.

The symptoms and when-to-seek-help boxes for each entry are your most useful tools in deciding whether you need emergency assistance, a visit to the doctor, or whether you can manage the problem at home. If you can't find your particular circumstances described in these boxes, call your nurse information service or doctor.

"Common Health Problems"—ones that are generally not life-threatening if diagnosed and treated early—follow, starting on page 115. These are organized similarly to "Major Health Concerns."

You'll also find two specialized sections—"Just for Women" (p. 207) and "Just for Men" (p. 229). As their names suggest, these sections deal with gender-specific illnesses and conditions.

Next comes a section on "Your Dental Health" (p. 241)—an important aspect of health that is often overlooked by older Americans. You'll find information on everything from how to recognize oral cancer to how to banish bad breath.

"On Your Mind" (p. 263) deals with depression, alcoholism, anxiety, and other mental health problems that often present great challenges to older people. In this section you also find tips for how to keep your brain active and your memory sharp as you age.

The management of medications—both prescription and non-prescription—is an important concern for older people. We have dedicated an entire section of the book, "Medication Matters" (p. 287), to the topic.

"Emergencies and First Aid" (p. 297) helps advise you on what to do during some of the most common medical emergencies. We strongly recommend that you read this section *before* a medical crisis arises.

In "Staying Safe" (p. 319) we've included detailed information about how to protect your safety and lower your risk of becoming a victim of an accident or a crime, including abuse and neglect.

Our last section, "Looking Ahead" (p. 333), offers advice on how you can plan for your retirement years and beyond. Such planning can help you stay independent longer.

Finally, we offer a "Resources" section (p. 341), which includes the telephone numbers, addresses, and Web sites of several dozen organizations you can contact for more information about health and aging.

In short, *Taking Care After 50* provides you with useful, practical information that will help make the prospect of aging well a reality.

Harvey Jay Cohen, MD

Prescription for Health

If I'd known I was going to live this long, I'd have taken better care of myself.
—Eubie Blake at age 100

It's *never* too late to start taking better care of ourselves! Study after study has shown that—no matter what our age—we can often keep and even improve our health simply by making a few changes in our daily lives. That's because many of the health problems associated with old age aren't due to age at all. They are due to unhealthful habits—things like smoking, overeating, not exercising, and drinking too much alcohol.

You can change those unhealthful habits—even if you've been practicing them for decades. Making such changes will not only help you prevent disease and injury, it can also help improve the quality of your life. Prevention is especially important because the older you become, the more at risk you are for certain diseases. And if you already have a chronic illness, developing more healthful habits may help slow the disease's progress. In some cases, it may even help reverse it.

You don't have to turn your life upside down to improve your health. Small lifestyle changes, such as taking a daily walk, adding more fruits and vegetables to your meals, and making sure you see your physician and dentist regularly, can reap major health rewards.

The important thing is that you start now. On the following pages you'll find "Eight Habits for Healthful Aging." They offer many good ideas for how you can begin to make more healthful choices in your life.

#1: Eat for Your Health

GOOD nutrition is good for your health, no matter what your age. Eating right can improve the quality of your life. It can give you more energy, for example, or help you sleep better at night. Eating healthful foods can also decrease the risk for certain diseases and delay the start of others. It may even help your body fight infection.

So what's a healthful diet? Here's what nutrition experts at the U.S. Department of Agriculture (USDA) say:

- Eat a variety of foods.
- Balance the food you eat with physical activity to maintain or improve your weight.
- Choose a diet with plenty of grain products, vegetables, and fruits.
- Choose a diet low in fat, saturated fat, and cholesterol.
- Choose a diet moderate in sugars.
- Choose a diet moderate in salt and sodium.
- If you drink alcoholic beverages, do so in moderation.

Did You Know?

The National Academy of Sciences estimates that 20 percent of all premature deaths in the United States could be avoided if people changed their eating habits. Their recommendation for a longer life: Eat less fat and more fruits, vegetables, legumes (dry beans and peas), and whole-grain breads and cereals.

To follow these guidelines, you don't have to overhaul your diet all at once. Start small. Make just one modest change in your daily diet. Try a slice of whole-wheat toast instead of white. Add some sliced fruit to your morning cereal. Switch from whole milk to 2 percent; then, a few weeks later, switch to 1 percent. Gradually make other changes. Over time, eating healthful foods will become a natural part of your life.

THE FOOD GUIDE PYRAMID
A Guide to Daily Food Choices

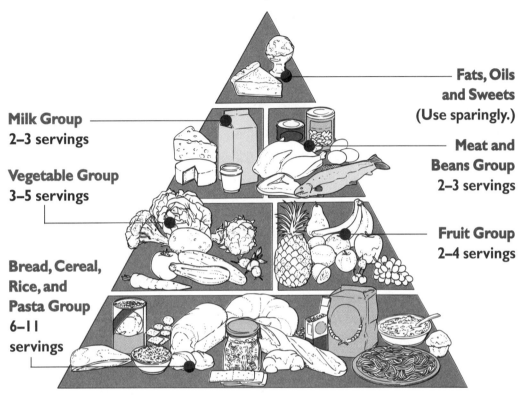

Fats, Oils and Sweets (Use sparingly.)

Milk Group
2–3 servings

Vegetable Group
3–5 servings

Meat and Beans Group
2–3 servings

Fruit Group
2–4 servings

Bread, Cereal, Rice, and Pasta Group
6–11 servings

The bulleted items below equal 1 serving.

Bread, Cereal, Rice, and Pasta Group
- 1 slice of bread
- 1 ounce of ready-to-eat cereal
- 1/2 cup of cooked cereal, rice, or pasta

Vegetable Group
- 1 cup of raw leafy vegetables
- 1/2 cup of other vegetables—cooked or chopped raw
- 3/4 cup of vegetable juice

Fruit Group
- 1 medium apple, banana, or orange
- 1/2 cup of chopped, cooked, or canned fruit
- 3/4 cup of fruit juice

Milk Group (milk, yogurt, and cheese)
- 1 cup of milk or yogurt
- 1 1/2 ounces of natural cheese
- 2 ounces of processed cheese

Meat and Beans Group (meat, poultry, fish, dry beans, eggs, and nuts)
- 2–3 ounces of cooked lean meat, poultry, or fish
- 1/2 cup of cooked dry beans, 1 egg, or 2 tablespoons of peanut butter count as 1 ounce of lean meat

The Food Guide Pyramid

Remember the four basic food groups? They have been replaced. Nutrition experts now recommend a new food guide: the Food Guide Pyramid. The Pyramid is designed to tell you at a glance how much of each kind of food you should eat. Specifically, it recommends that you

- choose most of your foods from the grain products group (6 to 11 servings daily), the vegetable group (3 to 5 servings daily), and the fruit group (2 to 4 servings daily);

- eat moderate amounts of foods from the milk group (2 to 3 servings daily) and the meat and beans group (2 to 3 servings daily); and

- choose sparingly foods that provide few nutrients and are high in fat and sugars.

The Pyramid offers a range of daily servings. The smaller number is for people who consume about 1,600 calories a day. The larger number is for those who consume about 2,800 calories a day. Experts generally recommend that older adults consume about 1,600 calories a day. If you are physically active, however, or need extra calories for medical reasons, you should eat additional servings. (For examples of serving sizes, see the Food Guide Pyramid, p. 3.)

Eat 5 a Day

Your mother was right: You should eat your fruits and vegetables. Research shows that these nutrient-packed foods can reduce the risk for **cancer**. That's because they are rich sources of vitamin A, vitamin C, fiber, and many other cancer-fighting compounds. But the benefits don't stop there. A diet rich in fruits and vegetables (and low in fats, particularly saturated fats) also lowers the risk for **coronary heart disease**, **high blood pressure**, and **diabetes**.

Health experts, including the National Cancer Institute and the American Heart Association, recommend that people of all ages eat *at least* 5 servings of fruits and vegetables each day. Be sure to eat a variety of fruits and vegetables. During the course of a day, try to include at least 1 serving each of a fruit or vegetable high in vitamin A, vitamin C, and fiber. Also, make sure you eat several servings of cruciferous vegetables a week. They have been found to contain particularly high amounts of natural cancer-fighting chemicals. (For good food sources of these nutrients, see chart opposite.)

GOOD SOURCES OF...

VITAMIN A	VITAMIN C	FIBER	CRUCIFEROUS VEGETABLES
Apricots	Bell peppers	Apple	Bok choy
Cantaloupe	Broccoli	Bran cereals	Broccoli
Carrots	Cantaloupe	Carrots	Brussels sprouts
Kale	Citrus fruits	Cooked beans	Cabbage
Mango	Leafy greens	Oatmeal	Cauliflower
Mustard greens	Potatoes	Peas	
Red peppers	Tomatoes	Strawberries	
		Whole-grain foods	

Source: National Cancer Institute

What Are Antioxidants and Why Do You Need Them?

As your body uses oxygen, it makes tiny substances known as *free radicals*. Free radicals attack healthy cells, weakening them. If left unchecked, they may contribute to heart damage, **cancer**, and cataracts. They may also weaken your immune system.

Antioxidants help protect healthy cells from the damage caused by free radicals. The best-known antioxidants are vitamin C, vitamin E, selenium, and carotenoids, which include beta-carotene, lycopene, and lutein. (See "Antioxidants," p. 6.)

Studies have shown that antioxidants are most effective when taken in combination. They also work better when taken with fiber. That's why it's best to get most of your antioxidants from your diet rather than from vitamin supplements. But if you can't get enough antioxidants from food alone, talk to your physician about taking them in supplement form.

ANTIOXIDANTS

	BENEFITS	GOOD SOURCES
Vitamin C	MAY PROTECT AGAINST: • Cataracts and other eye diseases MAY HELP: • Lower blood pressure and cholesterol • Prevent **stroke** and heart attacks	• Citrus fruits • Melons • Strawberries • Mangoes • Cruciferous vegetables
Vitamin E	MAY PROTECT AGAINST: • Certain forms of **cancer**, such as prostate and breast • Cardiovascular disease • **Vision problems**, such as macular degeneration and cataracts • Complications of **diabetes**, such as damage to small blood vessels • **Alzheimer's disease** • The stiffness associated with **arthritis**	• Fortified cereals • Whole grains • Wheat germ • Sunflower seeds • Nuts • Grain oils
Selenium	MAY PROTECT AGAINST: • **Arthritis** • Cardiovascular disease • **Cancer**	• Whole grains • Asparagus • Garlic • Eggs
Beta-carotene	MAY PROTECT AGAINST: • Prostate **cancer**	• Winter squash • Sweet potatoes
Lycopene	MAY PROTECT AGAINST: • Prostate and other kinds of **cancer**	• Tomatoes
Lutein	MAY HELP: • Lower the risk for developing the age-related eye disease known as macular degeneration	• Broccoli • Brussels sprouts • Spinach • Kale

Understanding Vitamins and Minerals

The recommendations for daily nutritional intake can be a helpful guideline.

RDAs—Recommended Dietary Allowances

RDAs mean the daily intake required to meet the nutritional needs of people in a particular group, for instance, people over age 50. RDAs are based on scientific evidence.

AIs—Adequate Intake

AIs refer to the goal for the daily intake of a nutrient for a particular group of people. AIs don't have scientific evidence.

Understanding vitamins, minerals and essential nutrients can be confusing. Also, nutritional information is continuously changing as scientists study it. Your best source of information is your own doctor.

If you take supplements, do so in moderation. They are usually safe at or below the RDA. But RDAs are

DIETARY INTAKE CHECKLIST

Here are daily essential nutrients for people ages 50 and older.

	MEN	WOMEN
Protein	63 g	50 g
Vitamin A[1]	900 mcg	700 mcg
Vitamin D[1]	10-15 mcg	10-15 mcg
Vitamin E	15 mg	15 mg
Vitamin K[1]	120 mcg	90 mcg
Vitamin C	90 mg	75 mg
Thiamin	1.2 mg	1.1 mg
Riboflavin	1.3 mg	1.1 mg
Niacin	16 mg	14 mg
Vitamin B_6	1.7 mg	1.5 mg
Folate (folic acid)	400 mcg	400 mcg
Vitamin B_{12}	2.4 mcg	2.4 mcg
Calcium[1]	1,200 mg	1,200 mg[2]
Phosphorus	700 mg	700 mg
Magnesium	420 mg	320 mg
Iron	8 mg	8 mg
Zinc	11 mg	8 mg
Iodine	150 mcg	150 mcg
Selenium	55 mcg	55 mcg

g = gram   mg = milligrams   mcg = micrograms

[1]These measurements are AIs. The rest are RDAs.

[2]A panel convened by the National Institutes of Health recommends that postmenopausal women who are not being treated with estrogen get 1,500 mg daily.

the *minimum* amounts required to prevent deficiencies.

Doses higher than the RDAs are sometimes recommended to prevent or treat certain diseases and conditions. Higher doses can be harmful, however. Take them only under the guidance of a physician or a registered dietitian.

Calcium Corner

Calcium helps keep blood pressure normal and thus may reduce the risk for **coronary heart disease**. When taken with vitamin D, calcium also may reduce the risk for colon **cancer**. Calcium is necessary for strong bones. It helps protect against the bone-thinning disease known as **osteoporosis**, which can lead to hip fractures and other bone problems. Hip fractures are the main reasons that older men and women enter assisted living facilities.

Yet an estimated 90 percent of all women and 60 percent of all men don't get enough calcium. The RDA for calcium for people over age 50 is 1,200 mg. A panel convened by the National Institutes of Health has recommended that postmenopausal women who are not taking estrogen supplements get 1,500 mg of calcium daily. Women are more prone than men to developing **osteoporosis**.

Self-Test

How Bone Smart Are You?

Do you eat 2 or more servings of milk, yogurt, cheese, or other calcium-fortified foods every day?
❏ Yes   ❏ No

Do you consistently check food labels for products that contain high calcium levels?
❏ Yes   ❏ No

Does your exercise routine include weight-lifting or weight-bearing activities?
❏ Yes   ❏ No

Do you regularly eat leafy green vegetables, calcium-enriched tofu, or fish with edible bones?
❏ Yes   ❏ No

Your Score

If you answered "Yes" to most of the above questions, you're on the right track for keeping your bones strong and meeting your calcium needs. Give yourself a pat on the back! If you answered "No" to many of the questions, there's a good chance that your bones are at risk.

Good food sources of calcium are low-fat dairy products, such as plain yogurt, part-skim ricotta and mozzarella cheeses, and skim milk. Other foods rich in calcium include collards, figs, tofu, calcium-enriched fruit juices, and pink salmon (canned with bones). If you don't get enough calcium from your diet, ask your physician if you should take a calcium supplement. The most effective supplements at reducing bone loss are calcium citrate and calcium gluconate. (Check the product label for these ingredients.) Some nutritionists recommend that you also take a vitamin D (400 to 800 IU) supplement. Vitamin D can help your body better absorb the calcium.

Water: The Forgotten Nutrient

As you get older, your body holds less water. Age can also hamper your ability to tell when you are thirsty. In addition, some medications can cause your body to lose water.

Now consider this: Not getting enough water can cause dizziness, put stress on your heart, and even result in a drop in blood pressure. It can also make you constipated.

It's recommended that you drink at least eight 8-ounce glasses of fluids each day. Choose fresh fruits and vegetables, soups, and juices. But don't count caffeinated coffee, tea, and sodas as part of your daily water quota. Caffeine acts as a diuretic and will actually cause your body to lose water.

The Scoop about Caffeine

Is caffeine—the stimulant found in coffee, tea, colas, chocolate, and some cold preparations—bad for your health? Yes and no, say scientists. Caffeine doesn't appear to increase the risk for **cancer**. And although drinking the equivalent of four or five cups of coffee a day can raise blood pressure and stress-related hormones in caffeine-sensitive people, caffeine doesn't appear to cause **coronary heart disease**, either—as long as coffee drinkers use filtered drip or instant coffee. (The filters and processing seem to remove any heart-harmful substances.)

Caffeine may be bad for your bones, however. Some research suggests that the more caffeine you consume, the more calcium is excreted in your urine. The result may be weaker bones. Other experts believe, however, that the scientific evidence does not support a link between caffeine consumption and **osteoporosis**. Still, if you are at risk for developing **osteoporosis**, you may want to eliminate or cut back the caffeine in your diet. At the very least, make sure you replace the lost calcium. Nutrition experts recommend that you drink an extra cup of nonfat or low-fat milk for each cup of coffee or two cans of caffeinated soda you consume.

Fill Up on Fiber

We used to call it *roughage* or *bulk*. Today we call it fiber. It's the material in plant cells that can't be fully digested. And it is an essential part of a healthful diet.

Fiber is found only in plant foods. There are two basic kinds of fiber: soluble and insoluble. Soluble fiber has been shown to help lower blood cholesterol. It may therefore help protect against **coronary heart disease**. Foods high in soluble fiber include oatmeal, beans, peas, rice, barley, citrus fruits, strawberries, and apples.

Insoluble fiber does not appear to lower blood pressure. But it helps bowels function properly. As a result, it reduces the risk for developing chronic **constipation**, **diverticulosis**, and **hemorrhoids**. Foods high in insoluble fiber include whole-grain breads and cereals, cabbage, beets, carrots, and Brussels sprouts.

Although recent research indicates that eating lots of high-fiber foods may not reduce the risk for colon cancer as much as previously thought, it may protect against other cancers. This may be because high-fiber foods tend to be rich in cancer-fighting nutrients.

FIBER

Food	Portion	Amount of Fiber (in grams)
Bran flake cereal	³/₄ cup	5.5
Pear, with skin	I medium	4.5
Kidney beans	¹/₂ cup	4.5
Potato, baked with skin	I medium	4.0
Oatmeal, cooked	¹/₂ cup	3.0
Apple, with skin	I medium	3.0
Whole-wheat bread	I slice	2.5
Orange	I medium	2.0

To get enough of both kinds of fiber, eat a variety of fruits, vegetables, and whole-grain breads and cereals. The American Dietetic Association recommends that all adults eat 20 to 35 grams of fiber a day. The typical American eats only half that amount. Older Americans often eat even less.

How do you know if you're eating enough fiber? The chart on p. 10 can give you a general idea of how much fiber you eat in an average day. Food labels also list dietary fiber. Read them carefully next time you shop.

Before You Take a Fiber Supplement

Studies have shown that certain fiber supplements can lower cholesterol levels in people who have high cholesterol. The supplements that were most studied contained guar gum, pectin, and psyllium. But before you run out to buy one of these supplements, consider the following:

- Getting your fiber from a supplement rather than food means you don't get all the healthful vitamins, minerals, and other nutrients that are also in fiber-rich foods. Many scientists believe that it is the interaction between fiber and these nutrients that makes high-fiber foods so good for you.

- Fiber supplements can result in unwanted side effects. Although it's uncommon, some people are allergic to psyllium, for example, and experience wheezing, chest tightness, or rashes after eating it. In rare cases, the reaction can be life-threatening.

The bottom line? A fiber supplement may be a good choice for you, but talk to your physician first.

The Whole Truth about Whole Grains

Whole grains are much more healthful than refined ones. They are loaded with the vitamins, minerals, fiber, and other nutrients that have been shown to help prevent **coronary heart disease**, **cancer**, and a host of other illnesses.

Refined grains, even "enriched ones," simply don't offer that level of protection. When a grain is refined, it is stripped of almost all its healthful nutrients. And "enriching" adds back only a few nutrients—several B vitamins and iron.

When it comes to shopping for whole grains, looks can be deceiving. A brown-colored bread, for example, is not necessarily a whole-wheat one. Nor is one that says it's made with "wheat flour." And crackers labeled "made with whole wheat" are actually made mostly with refined grain. So when shopping for whole grains, be alert—and adventurous! Here are some tips:

- When buying bread, make sure the *first* ingredient listed on the label is "whole-wheat flour." If the first ingredient is "wheat flour," "unbleached wheat flour," or "unbleached enriched wheat flour," put the bread back on the shelf. Those are just other names for "refined white flour."

- Don't be fooled by high-fiber "light" breads. They are all or mostly refined white flour. These breads may include processed fiber from peas or other foods. That added fiber may help prevent **constipation** and **diverticulitis**, but they don't include all the nutrients found in whole-wheat flour.

- Buy brown rice instead of white rice. You can now even find quick-cooking brown rice on most supermarket shelves.

- Look for whole-wheat pastas as well.

- Try cooking with other whole grains, such as amaranth, buckwheat groats (kasha), quinoa, or whole-grain bulgur.

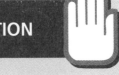

CAUTION

Increase the amount of fiber in your diet gradually. Your digestive system will need time to adapt. Also, be sure to drink lots of water—at least eight 8-ounce glasses a day. Eating too many high-fiber foods too quickly without increasing the amount of water you drink can cause stomach pains, gas, diarrhea, or **constipation**.

Some Facts about Fat

Everyone needs to eat *some* dietary fat to maintain good health. The problem is that most of us eat too much fat. High-fat diets have been linked to high blood cholesterol levels and an increased risk for **coronary heart disease**.

Fats come in three basic forms:

- Saturated (found in meat, dairy foods, and coconut and palm oils)

- Monounsaturated (found in olive, peanut, and canola oils)

- Polyunsaturated (found in high-fat fish and corn, cottonseed, safflower, soy, and sunflower oils)

Saturated fat raises blood cholesterol more than the other two forms of fat. In fact, some research indicates that a specific polyunsaturated fat found in fish (omega-3) may actually *decrease* the risk for **coronary heart disease**.

The American Heart Association recommends that no more than 30 percent of our daily calories come from fat. They also say that less than 10 percent of that fat should be in the form of saturated fat.

It's never too late to cut the fat and reap the health benefits. Read the following fat-reducing tips, then evaluate your total diet to see where you can make changes. Check food labels for fat content. The "Nutrition Facts" panel on most processed foods will tell you both the total and saturated fat content per serving.

Tips for Cutting the Fat

- Choose "lean" or "extra lean" cuts of meat. Trim all visible fat.

- Remove skin from poultry.

- Choose low-fat or nonfat milk, yogurt, sour cream, and cheeses.

- Season vegetables, meat, poultry, and fish with herbs, spices, lemon juice, and fat-free salad dressings instead of high-fat sauces.

- Reduce or eliminate from your diet high-fat processed meats, such as sausages, salami, and other cold cuts.

- Eat pasta, rice, and potatoes with low-fat sauces.

- Use fats and oils sparingly, both when cooking and at the table.

- Refrigerate soups and stews. Then, before eating, remove the fat that collects on the surface.

- Check nutrition labels; select foods low in fat and saturated fat.

Cut Down on Cholesterol, Too

Cholesterol is a fat that is found naturally in your body. It is needed for building cells, insulating nerves, and making hormones. But when too much cholesterol gets in your blood, your risk for developing **coronary heart disease** may increase. And that can lead to a heart attack or **stroke**.

Your body makes all the cholesterol you need. But you put extra cholesterol into your body every time you eat meat and dairy products. (Almost all other foods are naturally free of cholesterol.) The American Heart Association recommends that we limit our daily cholesterol intake to less than 300 mg.

How does that translate into what you eat? Here are some examples of cholesterol levels found in meats and seafood:

- 3.5 ounces liver, 400 mg

- 12 large shrimp, 130 mg

- 3.5 ounces extra-lean ground beef, 82 mg

- 3.5 ounces chicken breast meat, no skin, 73 mg

- 3.5 ounces perch, 36 mg

Egg yolks contain even more cholesterol than most meats—about 213 mg in each large egg. (Egg whites have no cholesterol.) But recent studies have found no long-term link between egg consumption and a higher risk for **coronary heart disease** or **stroke**—except among people with **diabetes**. The scientists who did these studies think that other nutrients in eggs, such as antioxidants, folate, B vitamins, and unsaturated fat, have a positive effect on the heart that more than offsets any negative impact from the eggs' cholesterol. More research is needed, however, to give eggs a totally clean bill of health. So talk to your physician before you start gobbling down eggs every morning for breakfast.

To eat less cholesterol, simply follow the fat-cutting tips (p. 13). Foods high in saturated fat also tend to be high in cholesterol. And if your physician tells you to cut back on eggs, try using egg whites or egg substitutes instead of whole eggs. Two egg whites can be used in place of one whole egg.

A Salty Controversy

Sodium is an important nutrient that is found naturally in foods. A little sodium in your diet is a good thing. But too much sodium *may* raise your blood pressure. **High blood pressure** is a leading cause of heart attacks and **stroke**.

Our most common source of sodium is salt (*sodium chloride*). Scientists disagree, however, about whether eating less salt can actually lower blood pressure and thus reduce the risk for **coronary heart disease** and **stroke**. Some studies have shown that cutting back on salt can lower blood pressure, particularly in people who already have **high blood pressure**. But other studies have shown that salt restriction has no such effect. The American Heart Association recommends that healthy Americans consume no more than 2,400 mg of sodium daily. That's the amount in about 1¼ teaspoons of salt.

So what should you do if you have **high blood pressure**? Talk to your physician. If you're told you need to cut back, read your food labels. You'll find that salt and sodium hide not just in salty foods like potato chips and hot dogs, but in a lot of processed foods, too.

How to Read a Food Label

It's a lot easier to choose healthful foods these days than it was in years past. Almost all packaged foods now contain easy-to-read labels. By reading those labels, you can find out not only what ingredients are in the product, but also specifics on fat, calories, sodium, and other nutrients.

If you're not already an expert food label reader, it's time you became one. Just look for the "Nutrition Facts" panel on the side or back of each food you buy. The label is loaded with helpful nutrition information about the food.

SAMPLE FOOD LABEL

Nutrition Facts		
Serving Size ½ cup (114g)		
Servings Per Container 4		
Amount Per Serving		
Calories 90	Calories from Fat 30	
		% Daily Value*
Total Fat 3g		**5%**
Saturated Fat 0g		**0%**
Cholesterol 0mg		**0%**
Sodium 300mg		**13%**
Total Carbohydrate 13g		**4%**
Dietary Fiber 3g		**12%**
Sugars 3g		
Protein 3g		
Vitamin A 80%	•	Vitamin C 60%
Calcium 4%	•	Iron 4%

* Percent Daily Values are based on a 2,000 calorie diet. Your daily values may be higher or lower depending on your calorie needs:

	Calories:	2,000	2,500
Total Fat	Less than	65g	80g
Sat Fat	Less than	20g	25g
Cholesterol	Less than	300mg	300mg
Sodium	Less than	2,400mg	2,400mg
Total Carbohydrate		300g	375g
Dietary Fiber		25g	30g

Calories per gram:
Fat 9 • Carbohydrate 4 • Protein 4

Source: U.S. Department of Agriculture

Here are the key things to look for when reading a food label:

1. Look at the serving size. It is about the same for similar items. So it's easy to compare the nutritional qualities of similar foods. *Warning:* A serving may be much smaller than you think!

2. Check the "Calories from Fat" number. Nutrition experts recommend that people get no more than 30 percent of the calories in their overall diet from fat.

3. Look at the column called "% Daily Value." It tells you if a food has large or small amounts of saturated fat, cholesterol, sodium, protein, fiber, sugars, vitamins, and minerals. Use this to compare different foods. And try to select as many low-fat or nonfat foods as possible—foods that have a 5 percent or less daily value for fat, saturated fat, and cholesterol.

Maintain a Healthy Weight

As we get older, most of us start gaining weight. And the weight gain goes on, decade after decade, pound after pound—until we often find ourselves overweight.

Being overweight can increase your risk for **high blood pressure**, **coronary heart disease**, **stroke**, **diabetes**, certain types of **cancer**, gout, and **gallstones**. It can also cause problems such as sleep apnea (interrupted breathing during sleep) and osteoarthritis. The more overweight you are, the more likely you are to have health problems.

If you are overweight, you should try to lose weight. Or, at the very least, you should avoid putting on any more pounds. Not sure whether your current weight puts you at risk? Check the chart on p. 18. Then talk to your physician.

The key to maintaining a healthy weight is simple. You've probably heard it many times before: Eat less and exercise more. That means making some changes to your diet. It also means finding ways to become more physically active. The changes don't have to be dramatic. Studies have shown that you can improve your health by losing as little as 10 to 20 pounds.

Here are some tips for safe, healthy weight loss:

- Commit yourself to making permanent changes in your diet.

- Increase your daily physical activity.

- Make sure you eat at least 1,200 calories each day. You should never go on a diet of less than 1,200 calories without your physician's supervision.

- Eat a variety of foods that are low in calories and high in nutrients.

- Eat less fat and fewer high-fat foods. But remember that low fat does not always mean low in calories.

- Eat smaller portions.

- Eat more vegetables and fruits—but don't drench them with fatty or sugary sauces or toppings.

- Eat whole-grain pasta, rice, breads, and cereals. Again, don't top them with fatty or sugary sauces or spreads.

- Eat less sugar and fewer sweets (such as candy, cookies, cakes, and soda).

- Drink little or no alcohol.

If You Need to Gain Weight

Being too thin can be unhealthy, too. It may mean you're not getting all the nutrients you need. As a result, you may develop health problems. Also, if you've lost weight, you may have lost muscle. Weakened muscles can increase your risk for falls and bone fractures.

Be sure to bring any sudden weight loss to the attention of your physician. A drop in pounds can be a sign of physical illness or of **depression**. You should also let your physician know if you've been eating less or skipping meals. After evaluating your physical health, your physician may refer you to a nutritionist to help you regain your appetite and those lost pounds.

Here are some easy ways to increase calories:

- Eat something every three hours. It can be a small meal or a simple snack. Want some easy-to-prepare snack ideas? Try peanut butter and crackers, a fruit muffin, custards, or puddings.

- Drink fruit juices. They are rich in calories. One cup of orange juice, for example, has 110 calories. You'd have to eat almost two whole oranges to get that same amount.

- Add 1 to 2 tablespoons of nonfat dry milk to soups and sauces.

Did You Know?

If you are a woman and your waist measures more than 35 inches, or if you are a man and your waist measures more than 40 inches, you are more likely to develop **high blood pressure**, **diabetes**, **coronary heart disease**, and certain types of **cancer**. Talk to your physician about the health risks of your weight.

- Try not to begin a meal with soup or a beverage. They may fill you up and keep you from eating higher-calorie foods.
- Add raisins or other dried fruit to your morning cereal.

ARE YOU OVERWEIGHT?

Use the weight-for-height chart below to see if you're overweight. Find your height in the left-hand column and move across the row to find your weight. If your weight falls within the moderate to severe overweight range on the chart, you are more likely to have health problems.

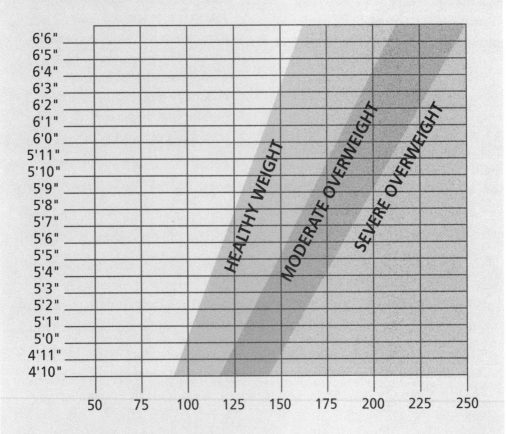

Source: U.S. Department of Agriculture

Do You Have Trouble Chewing or Swallowing?

It's not unusual for older people to have chewing or swallowing problems that make it difficult to eat a healthful, well-balanced diet. Fortunately these problems can be corrected.

If you have trouble chewing, see your dentist. You may have broken or improperly fitted bridges or dentures. Until your teeth are fixed, cut your food into small, bite-size pieces. Correcting your teeth may also make it easier to swallow. But if the problem persists, ask your physician for a referral to a speech therapist. The therapist will give you a swallowing test and help you correct any problem. Meanwhile buy soft, easy-to-swallow foods, such as yogurt, soups, and cooked fruits, vegetables, and whole-grain cereals.

For more information about dental care and problems, see pp. 241-259.

Tips for Preventing Food-Borne Illness

Salmonella. E. coli. Shigella. These are just a few of the microbes that can cause food-borne illnesses, better known as food poisoning. Each year food-borne illnesses strike an estimated 6 to 33 million people in the United States. The symptoms include vomiting, diarrhea, and stomach cramps. Most adults usually recover within a day or two. But for some people—the very young, the elderly, and those with an impaired immune system (such as people with **cancer** and **diabetes**)—a food-borne illness can be more serious, even life-threatening. About 9,000 Americans die from these illnesses each year.

Did You Know?

As we age, our need for calories may decline by as much as 25 percent. But our vitamin and mineral requirements stay the same—or in some cases even increase. As a result, we have to make sure we do two things. First, we need to pay attention to how many calories we take in to make sure we don't put on extra, unhealthful pounds. Second, we need to make sure the foods we eat are packed with all the nutrients we need.

Most food-borne illnesses are preventable. Here are some steps you can take to lower your risk:

- Make the grocery store your last stop on your list of errands; get cold foods home to a refrigerator or freezer as quickly as possible.

- Buy only pasteurized dairy products and fruit juices.

- Wash your hands in warm soapy water before and after handling food, especially fresh whole fruits and vegetables and raw meat, poultry, fish, and eggs. Also, thoroughly wash cooking utensils and surfaces before using them again for other foods.

- Rinse raw fruits and vegetables in warm water. If necessary, use a small scrub brush to remove surface dirt.

- Thoroughly cook all meat, poultry, and seafood (especially shellfish).

- Cover and store leftover cooked food in the refrigerator as soon as possible.

- Keep your refrigerator at no higher than 40 degrees F and your freezer at 0 degrees F.

- Reheat all leftovers until they are steaming hot.

#2: Stay Active

MOVE more! It will improve your health. In fact, the older you are the more you need to stay physically active. Exercise is good for your heart, lungs, muscles, joints, bones, and even your skin. It slows the aging process. It also reduces the risk for many diseases associated with aging, including **coronary heart disease**, **cancer**, **diabetes**, and **osteoporosis**.

But it's not just your physical health that will benefit when you get out of your chair and start moving. Being physically active has been shown to help relieve symptoms of **depression** and **anxiety**. It can reduce stress and tension. It can also help you keep your mind sharp.

So keep moving. You'll enjoy a higher quality of life and more independence as you age. Everyday activities—carrying groceries, lifting a grandchild, gardening, and even driving a car—may be much easier. And being active will also give you greater opportunities to meet new people as well as stay in touch with old friends.

A Well-Rounded Exercise Program

As you plan an exercise program, you'll want to make sure it has three key elements: aerobic activity, strength exercises, and stretching.

Aerobic Activity

An aerobic activity is one that causes you to breathe harder and your heart to beat faster than usual for a prolonged period of time. If done regularly, aerobic exercise will strengthen your heart and lungs.

When we hear the term *aerobic exercise* most of us think of activities such as walking, running, swimming, bicycling, and aerobic exercise classes. (Many health clubs now offer aerobic classes designed specifically for older adults.) But if none of these activities appeal to you, don't worry. Health experts now say that even moderately intense activities, if done every day, can provide some long-term health benefits.

What is a moderately intense activity? Almost anything that gets you moving.

15 REASONS TO STAY ACTIVE PAST 50

Studies have shown that regular physical exercise can help you

1. slow the aging process and help you look and feel better.
2. increase your stamina and energy.
3. keep your weight within a healthy range.
4. keep your mind sharp as you age.
5. lower your blood pressure and your resting heart rate; as a result, your heart won't have to work as hard.
6. reduce your risk for developing **diabetes**.
7. reduce your risk for developing some kinds of **cancer**.
8. strengthen your bones to protect against **osteoporosis**.
9. strengthen your muscles, giving you more endurance.
10. keep joints, tendons, and ligaments more flexible, making it easier for you to move.
11. improve your digestion and elimination.
12. increase your sense of balance and agility, thus reducing your risk for injuring yourself from a fall or accident.
13. decrease stress, tension, and **anxiety**, thus improving your sense of well-being.
14. sleep better.
15. stay independent longer.

Such activities include walking, gardening, raking leaves, climbing stairs, moderate to heavy housework, and dancing.

Even the walking you do while shopping at the mall counts! ("Water walking" in a pool is a great alternative for people with **arthritis**.)

Here are the two key points to remember:

- Aim for 30 minutes of activity. You don't have to do the 30 minutes all at once, however. You could split it up, for example, into three 10-minute segments.

- The activity should be done on most, and preferably all, days of the week.

Strength Exercises

People who are inactive lose about 3 to 5 percent of their muscle fiber every decade after age 30. So by the time they're 60, they've lost 15 percent of their muscle fiber!

Strength exercises (also known as *weight lifting* or *resistance training*) can help you build and maintain your muscles. They can also help you keep your bones and joints healthy. Studies have shown that older adults who lift small amounts of weight regularly are less likely to fall and break a bone. And although strength exercises won't cure **arthritis**, they can help lessen its symptoms.

Strength exercises also increase your metabolism, which can make it easier to keep your weight and blood sugar in check. That's important because obesity and **diabetes** are major health problems for older adults.

You don't have to build huge mounds of muscle on your arms and legs to start reaping these health benefits. Even a very small increase in muscle mass can make a big difference, especially in people who have lost a lot of muscle. And you don't have to join a health club or buy fancy equipment to do these kinds of exercises. You can do simple strength training using household items, such as soup cans. Start by lifting light weights—1 to 2 pounds. To avoid injury, have a trained instructor teach you how to work with weights. Community and senior centers often offer strength-training classes. Look for one near you.

Here are some points to remember:

- Do strengthening exercises for both upper and lower body.

- Do the exercises for 30 to 40 minutes at least two or three times each week.

- Don't exercise the same muscles two days in a row. Give them time to recover.

CAUTION

You should consult with your physician before starting a vigorous exercise activity. Strenuous activity could be a problem for people with "hidden" **coronary heart disease**—that is, people who have heart disease but don't know it because they have no symptoms.

But remember: Most older adults—no matter what their age or health condition—do fine when they increase their physical activity. In fact, regular exercise is usually just what the doctor ordered!

Stretching

Stretching can improve your flexibility, making it easier for you to reach, turn, and move about. When you're flexible you're also less likely to lose your balance and fall. Falls are one of the leading causes of injuries in older adults. Regular stretching can also help reduce some of the stiffness and pain of **arthritis**. It's also very relaxing and can help you sleep better.

Here are some points to remember about stretching:

- You can do simple stretching exercises throughout the day. But if possible, try to set aside a regular "stretching" time. Evening is a great time to stretch because your muscles are already warmed up from the day's activities. Stretching in the evening can also help you fall asleep.

- Do stretching exercises for 5 to 15 minutes, preferably every day.

- Be sure to stretch muscles in all parts of your body.

Some Tips for Getting Started—and Staying Active

- Start slowly. If you start out too fast, you may get discouraged and give up. Or you may get injured.

- Choose activities that you enjoy.

- Begin with a modest goal. For example, try adding a short after-dinner walk to your daily schedule. Start with a 5- to 10-minute walk, then gradually work up to 30 minutes.

Did You Know?

You're probably aware of the Surgeon General's report that warns people about the health dangers of cigarette smoke. What you may not know is that the Surgeon General also issued a report warning people—including older adults—about another major risk to their health: physical inactivity.

- Ask someone to exercise with you. Many people find it easier to stay active when they have company.

- Wear comfortable clothing. Make sure your footwear fits properly.

- Set an exercise goal and reward yourself when you reach that goal. Then set a new goal.

- Schedule your exercise sessions. Think of them as appointments. If possible, try to schedule them for the same time each day. You are more likely to stick to an exercise program when you have set aside a regular time for it.

- Keep track of what you do and how you are progressing. Be patient! It may be several weeks before you start noticing any changes in how you look or feel.

A Few Strength Exercises

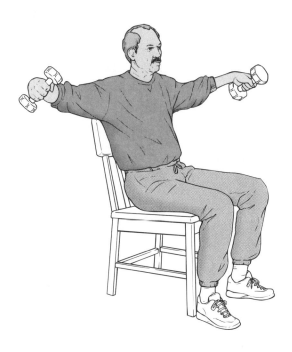

Arm Raise: Strengthens shoulders.

1. Sit in a chair.

2. Put your feet flat on the floor, keeping them even with your shoulders.

3. Put your arms straight down at your sides, palms inward.

4. Slowly raise both arms to the side, shoulder height.

5. Hold the position for a slow count of 10.

6. Slowly lower your arms to your sides.

7. Repeat 8 to 15 times. (You can intensify this exercise by using light hand held weights.)

Hip Flex: Strengthens thigh and hip muscles.

1. Stand straight, holding on to a tall, stable object (such as the back of a chair) for balance.
2. Slowly lift one knee toward your chest, without bending your waist or hips.
3. Hold the position for a slow count of 10.
4. Slowly lower your knee all the way down.
5. Repeat with the other leg.
6. Repeat 8 to 15 times with each leg.

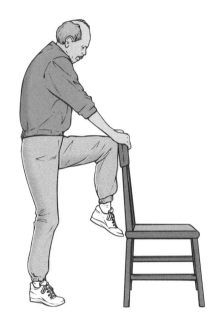

A Few Stretching Exercises

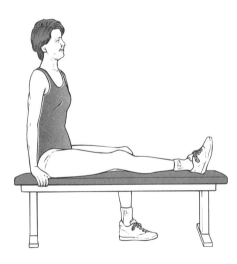

Hamstrings: Stretches muscles in back of thigh.

1. Sit sideways on a bench or other hard surface (such as two chairs placed side by side).
2. Keep one leg stretched out on the bench.
3. Place the other leg off the bench, with the foot flat on the floor.
4. Straighten your back.
5. Lean forward from the hips (not the waist) until you feel stretching in the leg on the bench, keeping your back and shoulders straight. *Caution:* Omit this step if you have had a hip replacement, unless your physician approves.
6. Hold the position for a slow count of 10.
7. Repeat with the other leg.
8. Repeat 3 to 5 times on each side.

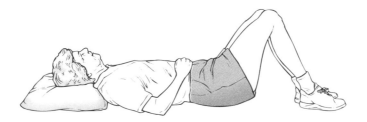

Double Hip Rotation: Stretches the outer muscles of hips and thighs.

Caution: Don't do this exercise if you have had a hip replacement, unless your physician approves.

1. Lie on your back, with your knees bent and your feet flat on the floor.

2. Keep your knees together and your shoulders touching the floor at all times; lower your legs to one side.

3. Hold the position for a slow count of 10.

4. Return your legs to the upright position.

5. Repeat on the other side.

6. Repeat 3 to 5 times on each side.

Shoulder Rotation: Stretches the shoulder muscles.

1. Lie flat on the floor, with a pillow under your head.

2. Stretch your arms out to the side.

3. Keep your shoulders flat on the floor throughout.

4. Bend your elbows to crook lower arms downward, at right angle.

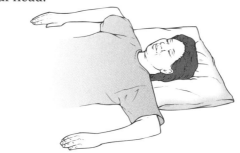

5. Hold this for a slow count of 10.

6. Bend your elbows to crook lower arms upward, at right angle.

7. Hold this position for a slow count of 10.

8. Repeat 3 to 5 times.

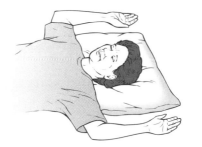

Source: National Institute on Aging

Everyday Ways to Become More Active

- When shopping or doing errands, park your car in the farthest corner of the parking lot and walk to the building—unless you are concerned about safety.

- Take the stairs whenever possible.

- Put on some music in the evening, clear some floor space, and dance!

- Get in the habit of doing simple neck and shoulder stretches after you've been sitting in a chair for a while.

- Take your dog for longer walks.

- Do chores that move your arms and legs, such as reorganizing your closet or washing the car.

- Put your television-watching time to good use. Do your stretching and strength exercises in front of the TV. Or invest in a stationary bike and cycle your way through your favorite show.

#3: Quit Smoking

SMOKING cigarettes is the leading preventable cause of premature death in the United States. Smoking kills more than 400,000 people every year. It also lessens the quality of life for many others. That's because smoking contributes to a long and frightening list of diseases, including **coronary heart disease**, **stroke**, emphysema, **osteoporosis**, and several kinds of **cancer**. Smokers, on average, die nearly seven years earlier than nonsmokers.

If you smoke, you're also harming the health of your loved ones and of others around you. It is estimated that about 3,000 nonsmokers die each year from lung **cancer** caused by secondhand smoke or smoke from other people's cigarettes. Even pets are at risk. Researchers have found that secondhand smoke increases the risk for lung cancer in dogs.

So for your health and the health of the people (and animals!) you love, stop smoking. No matter how old you are or how long you've been smoking or how many times you've tried to quit in the past, you can kick the habit for good. Ask your physician for a referral to a stop-smoking program in your area. Or call your local chapter of the American Heart Association, the American Lung Association, or the American Cancer Society.

Great Reasons to Quit Smoking

Although much depends on how long and how heavily you have smoked, you can expect to experience some, and perhaps all, of the following benefits after you quit:

- Your sense of taste and smell will return.

- Your smoker's cough will go away.

- You'll have more energy.

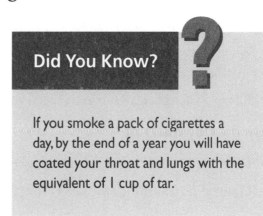

Did You Know?

If you smoke a pack of cigarettes a day, by the end of a year you will have coated your throat and lungs with the equivalent of 1 cup of tar.

- You'll breathe easier.

- You'll digest your food more easily.

- Your hair, clothes, and skin will smell better. So will your home.

- You'll look better. Your teeth and fingers will no longer be stained from nicotine, and your skin will look healthier.

- You'll have more money. (Multiply the cost of your daily supply of nicotine by 365. You may be shocked to find out just how much you spend on tobacco each year.)

- You'll live longer. That's because you'll be less at risk for developing **coronary heart disease**, lung disease, **cancer**, and other life-threatening illnesses.

- You'll make your loved ones happy. They want you to live a long and healthy life.

- You'll feel better about yourself.

Quitting Tips

Quitting smoking is not easy. Still, it *can* be done, no matter how long you've been smoking. Here are some tips from the National Cancer Institute.

Getting Ready to Quit

- Set a date for quitting. If possible, have a friend quit smoking with you.

- Notice when and why you smoke. Notice things in your daily life that you often do while smoking (such as drinking your morning cup of coffee or driving a car).

- Change your smoking routines: Keep your cigarettes in a different place. Smoke with your other hand. Don't do anything else when smoking. Think about how you feel when you smoke.

- Smoke only in certain places, such as outdoors.

- When you want a cigarette, wait a few minutes. Try to think of something to do instead of smoking; you might chew gum or drink a glass of water.

- Buy one pack of cigarettes at a time. Switch to a brand of cigarettes you don't like.

On the Day You Quit

- Get rid of all your cigarettes. Put away your ashtrays.

- Change your morning routine to avoid that first cigarette. Stay busy.

- When you get the urge to smoke, do something else instead. Carry other things to put in your mouth, such as gum, hard candy, or a toothpick.
- Reward yourself at the end of the day for not smoking. See a movie or go out and enjoy your favorite meal.

Staying Away from Tobacco

- Don't worry if you're sleepier or more short-tempered than usual; these feelings will pass.
- Try to exercise—take walks or ride a bike. It will help distract you and cut the cravings.
- Consider the positive things about quitting, such as how much you like yourself as a nonsmoker, the health benefits for you and your family, and the example you set for others around you. A positive attitude will help you through the tough times.
- When you feel tense, try to keep busy, think about ways to solve the problem, tell yourself that smoking won't make it any better, and go do something else.
- Eat regular meals. Hunger is sometimes mistaken for the desire to smoke.
- Start a money jar with the money you save by not buying cigarettes. Count it when you feel a craving.
- Let others know that you have quit smoking—most people will support you. Many of your smoking friends may want to know how you quit. It's good to talk to others about your quitting.
- If you slip and smoke, don't be discouraged. Many former smokers tried to stop several times before they finally succeeded. Quit again.

Patches, Gums, Sprays, and Other Quitting Aids

In recent years new products have come on the market that can help you kick your nicotine habit. Several brands of nicotine patches and nicotine gum are available over the counter. A nicotine nasal spray and inhaler, as well as a non-nicotine medication, are currently available by prescription. These products can help relieve the withdrawal symptoms that you'll experience when you quit smoking.

Nicotine patches, gum, and medications tend to be most effective when combined with a behavior change program. Your physician can advise you on which product and which program can best help you.

Throw Away Your Cigars, Pipes, and Chewing Tobacco, Too

Cigars, pipes, and chewing tobacco are not safe alternatives to cigarettes. Using these products puts you at greater risk for dying from cancers of the mouth, larynx, and esophagus than a nonsmoker. Smoking cigars or pipes also increases your risk for developing lung **cancer**.

THE HEALTH REWARDS OF QUITTING

Within hours of stopping smoking your body will start to heal itself. Here's what you can expect:

8 to 12 hours after quitting: The levels of nicotine and carbon monoxide in your blood drop by half. Oxygen levels return to normal (unless you have a chronic lung disease).

24 hours after quitting: All carbon monoxide is out of your body. Your lungs start to get rid of mucus and other smoking debris. Your smoker's hack begins to disappear.

48 hours after quitting: All nicotine is out of your body. Your sense of smell and taste improves. Breathing becomes easier. You begin to feel that you have more energy.

2 to 12 weeks after quitting: Your circulation improves.

3 to 9 months after quitting: Your lungs are now working about 10 percent more efficiently than when you were smoking. Your coughing and breathing problems continue to improve.

5 years after quitting: Your risk for heart attack drops to half that of a smoker.

10 years after quitting: Your risk for lung **cancer** drops to half that of a smoker. Your risk for heart attack falls to that of someone who has never smoked.

#4: If You Drink Alcohol, Do So Wisely

As you age, your body becomes less able to absorb and get rid of alcohol. The alcohol you drink, therefore, is going to have more of an impact on your body—and on your behavior—than it did when you were younger.

To begin with, alcohol slows brain activity. This can affect your alertness, judgment, coordination, and reaction time. Older people are already at greater risk for falling. Drinking only increases that risk, as well as the risk for other kinds of accidents.

Alcohol can also make it more difficult to diagnose certain medical problems associated with aging. For example, alcohol can cause changes in the heart and blood vessels that dull the pain associated with a heart attack. It can also cause forgetfulness and confusion—symptoms that can be mistaken for **Alzheimer's disease**.

In addition, mixing alcohol with over-the-counter or prescription drugs can be dangerous. The risk is especially great for older people, who tend to take many medications.

If you drink alcohol, it's important that you do so wisely. Public health officials recommend that women limit their alcoholic consumption to one drink and men to one or two drinks per day. A drink is

- 12 ounces of beer;
- 5 ounces of wine;
- 1.5 ounces of 80-proof distilled spirits.

Did You Know?

Drinking purple grape juice may be just as healthful for your heart as drinking red wine. That's because both red wine and purple grape juice contain resveratrol, a natural anti-oxidant found in the skin of grapes.

Studies have shown that resveratrol helps keep blood cells from clotting together and blocking arteries.

But for some older people, even that amount may be too much. If you think alcohol is having a negative effect on your health, stop drinking and talk to your physician. The decision on how much, if any, alcohol you should drink is best made in consultation with your physician.

If you find that you *can't* stop drinking, you may have an alcohol problem. You'll find more information on alcohol abuse, including how to recognize it, on pp. 266-270.

Alcohol, Coronary Heart Disease, and Cancer

Studies have shown that moderate alcohol drinking can lower the risk for **coronary heart disease**. What is moderate drinking? For men, it's one to two drinks per day. For women, it's one drink per day.

You should also know, however, that drinking alcohol—especially in combination with smoking or chewing tobacco—can increase your risk for **cancer** of the mouth and esophagus. This risk may begin with as few as two drinks a day. Alcohol may also increase the risk for **breast cancer**—and with just a few drinks per week.

For men over age 50 and women over age 60 the cardiovascular benefits of moderate alcohol consumption may outweigh the risks for **cancer**. Still, health officials don't advise nondrinkers to start drinking.

The Dangers of Mixing Alcohol and Medications

Mixing alcohol and medications can be risky. This is true for over-the-counter as well as prescription drugs. Alcohol can keep some drugs from doing what they are supposed to, whether it's repairing the body or preventing an illness. Alcohol can also make some drugs *too* effective, causing unwanted and even life-threatening side effects.

If you drink alcohol, always ask your physician or pharmacist about how a medication you take reacts with alcohol. A list of some of the more common alcohol-drug interactions can be found on the opposite page.

MEDICATION	WHEN COMBINED WITH ALCOHOL...
Antibiotics	May cause nausea, vomiting, **headaches**, and possibly convulsions.
Antidepressants	May increase the sedative effect of the drugs; with some antidepressants, may cause blood pressure to go dangerously high.
Antidiabetic medications	May make the drugs less effective or sometimes too effective; may also cause nausea and **headaches**.
Antihistamines	May increase the sedative effect of the drugs, causing dizziness or drowsiness.
Barbiturates	May make the drugs less effective; in some cases may lead to coma or death.
Cardiovascular medications	May make the drugs less effective; may also cause dizziness.
Narcotic pain relievers	May increase the sedative effect of the drugs, which increases the risk for death by overdose.
Non-narcotic pain relievers	May increase the risk for stomach bleeding; may cause liver damage.
Sedatives and hypnotics ("sleeping pills")	May cause severe drowsiness, increasing the risk for falling and other accidents.

#5: Reduce Stress

STRESS is your body's natural reaction to any demand put on it. The reaction is automatic and immediate. Your heart starts beating faster and your blood pressure shoots up. More blood flows to your brain, heart, and muscles and less to your skin, digestive tract, kidneys, and liver. Your muscles tense and you become more alert.

All these reactions are meant to protect your body. They are part of the "fight or flight response"—nature's way of giving you the energy to either fight or flee from danger. But if the stress is repeated too often or if it continues without relief, it can have serious effects.

Too much stress can seriously damage your physical health. Stress can cause a host of relatively minor health problems, such as **back and neck problems**, **headaches**, and **indigestion**. It can weaken your immune system, so you'll catch more **colds** and other infections. Stress can also lead to potentially life-threatening diseases, such as **high blood pressure** and **coronary heart disease**.

Stress can take a toll on your emotional health as well. It can cause you to become more anxious, nervous, and depressed. You may have trouble sleeping. Increased irritability and sudden flashes of anger are also symptoms of stress. Many people also lose their ability to put events and situations in perspective—and their sense of humor.

Mental capabilities often diminish under stress. You may have trouble remembering or concentrating. Many people under stress also experience behavioral changes. Some people develop nervous habits, such as nail biting or foot tapping. Or they make unhealthful lifestyle changes, such as overeating, smoking, or drinking too much alcohol.

Such symptoms affect not only our personal health and well-being, but also our relationships with the people around us. When you are under stress, the people you care about suffer as well.

Sorting the Good from the Bad

Not all stress is bad. In fact, without stress our lives would be very dull. Stress causes tension, but often with pleasurable results. Hosting a party, for example, can be stressful but also a lot of fun. So can watching your favorite sports team compete in a close game. A little bit of stress helps many of us be more productive. And when we get things done we tend to feel better about ourselves.

Each of us reacts to stress in a different way. That's because it's not a particular event or situation that's stressful, but how we perceive it. What is stressful for one person may not be stressful for someone else. Some people, for example, enjoy speaking before an audience. Others find it very stressful. Some people find driving a car relaxing. Others tense up behind the wheel.

Did You Know?

Pets can be great stress-reducers. Studies have shown that just being around animals can lower stress and anxiety for many people.

The key, then, is to learn how to recognize and reduce the *bad* stress in your life. One way of doing this is to conduct a personal stress audit. List the things in your life that create feelings of stress. Then write down what steps you can take to lessen that stress. Concentrate on the things you can change—and try to avoid the others.

Here are some examples of types of *stressors*, or things that can trigger stress.

- Environmental: Noise, bright lights, excessive heat or cold.

- Social: Rudeness or aggressiveness from another person.

- Organizational: Rules and regulations, filling out excessive paperwork, meeting deadlines.

- Major life events: Death or illness of a loved one, divorce, retirement.

- Daily hassles: Misplacing keys, driving in heavy traffic, waiting in a long line.

- Lifestyle choices: Trying to do "too much," drinking caffeinated or alcoholic beverages, not getting enough sleep.

Tips for Coping with Stress

- Cut down on caffeine. It's a stimulant and can make you feel more stressed. Also, limit alcohol and don't smoke.

- Eat healthful foods. When you're under stress, your body needs all the vitamins and minerals it can get.

- Exercise regularly. Physical activity releases chemicals in your body that can help relieve symptoms of **anxiety** and **depression**.

- Get enough sleep.

Self-Test

Are You Under Too Much Stress?

Do minor problems and disappointments upset you excessively?
☐ Yes   ☐ No

Do the small pleasures of life fail to satisfy you?
☐ Yes   ☐ No

Are you unable to stop thinking of your worries?
☐ Yes   ☐ No

Do you feel inadequate or suffer from self-doubt?
☐ Yes   ☐ No

Are you constantly tired?
☐ Yes   ☐ No

Do you experience flashes of anger over situations that never bothered you before?
☐ Yes   ☐ No

Have you noticed a change in sleeping or eating patterns?
☐ Yes   ☐ No

Do you suffer from chronic pain, headaches, or backaches?
☐ Yes   ☐ No

If most of your answers were "Yes," you may be under too much stress. You should find better ways of reducing or managing the stress in your life.

Source: National Mental Health Association

- Take time to relax every day. Choose a method of relaxation that you enjoy. It can be a traditional relaxation technique such as yoga or meditation. Or it can be something as simple as setting aside quiet time to read or listen to music.

- Get organized. Get in the practice of making lists. Learn how to prioritize—and how to say no.

- Communicate. Let the people around you know that you are going through a particularly stressful period. They will be more understanding of your mood changes and may offer to help you manage some of your stressors. Also, talking to someone may help you find solutions to some of your worries.

- Try to remain optimistic. Push away gloomy thoughts as much as possible. Seek out other optimistic people.

- Keep your sense of humor. If you feel it fading, "jump-start" it by renting a funny video or reading a humorous book.

When to Seek Professional Help

If your stress is significantly interfering with your daily life and if self-care measures aren't working, you may want to consider professional help. Talk to your physician, clergy or spiritual adviser, or local mental health association. They can refer you to a psychiatrist, psychologist, social worker, or other qualified counselor.

#6: Get Regular Checkups and Health Screenings

Y EARS ago people went to a doctor only when they were sick or injured. Today health experts recommend that all of us see our physicians regularly—even when we are feeling well. Such visits are called preventive checkups. They can help detect problems early on, when treatment is likely to be most effective. They also can help keep health problems from developing in the first place.

At each checkup you may undergo routine tests (also known as *screenings*). These tests range from having your height and weight measured to examining your colon for colorectal **cancer**. Not every health screening test will be done at every checkup. Your physician will tell you when you are due for a particular screening.

How frequently you should have preventive checkups will depend on your age and medical condition. Talk to your physician about how often you should come in for checkups and screenings. (For information on how to prepare for a visit to your physician, see pp. 44-47.)

If You Are Planning a Trip Abroad

Before traveling abroad, ask your physician what immunizations or medications, if any, you may need.

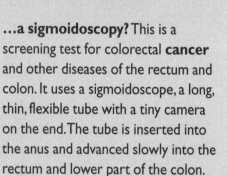

What is...?

...a sigmoidoscopy? This is a screening test for colorectal **cancer** and other diseases of the rectum and colon. It uses a sigmoidoscope, a long, thin, flexible tube with a tiny camera on the end. The tube is inserted into the anus and advanced slowly into the rectum and lower part of the colon. Your physician will use it to look for cancer and polyps that may be an early sign of **cancer**.

...a fecal occult blood test? This test uses a stool sample to check for traces of blood, which can be a sign of colorectal **cancer**.

RECOMMENDED PREVENTIVE HEALTH SCREENINGS—AND WHEN YOU SHOULD HAVE THEM

Screening	Ages 50-64	Ages 65 and Older
Height/weight	Periodically	Periodically*
Blood pressure	Periodically	Periodically*
Total blood cholesterol	Periodically	
Fecal occult blood test	Annually	Annually*
Sigmoidoscopy	Every 3 to 5 years	Every 3 to 5 years
Clinical breast exam (women)	Every 1 to 2 years	Every 1 to 2 years until age 69*
Mammogram (women)	Every 1 to 2 years	Every 1 to 2 years until age 69*
Papanicolaou (Pap) test (women)	Every 1 to 3 years for sexually active females who have not had a hysterectomy	Every 2 to 3 years for sexually active females who have not had a hysterectomy; consider discontinuing if previous regular screenings were normal*
Vision screening	Annually	Annually
Hearing assessment	Periodically	Periodically

Source: U.S. Preventive Services Task Force and Optum

* Frequency and tests beyond age 69 should be discussed with your physician.

Note: Other authorities' recommendations may differ from these. People at high risk for particular diseases or conditions may need additional screenings. Check with your physician.

IMMUNIZATIONS: NOT FOR KIDS ONLY

Immunizations are not just for children. Adults also need to be vaccinated from time to time. In fact, some immunizations are more important for older adults than for children. Each year thousands of older people die needlessly from illnesses that could have been prevented with a simple shot.

Here are the recommended immunizations for people aged 50 and older.

Immunization	Ages 50-64	Ages 65 and Older
Influenza (the "flu")	Annually for people at high risk*	Annually
Pneumococcal disease (including **pneumonia** and meningitis)	Once for people with chronic illness*	Once for all people whose immune systems have not been compromised*
Tetanus and diphtheria	Boosters every 10 years, or as recommended†	Boosters every 10 years, or as recommended†

Source: U.S. Preventive Services Task Force and Optum
* Check with your physician.
† Frequency should be discussed with your physician.

Vaccines against certain diseases, such as hepatitis A, yellow fever, and typhoid fever, are recommended for people traveling to various areas of the world. Some immunizations require a series of shots. It is best to contact your physician early—at least six months before your trip, if possible.

Get Regular Dental Checkups, Too

You should see a dentist every six months to a year for an exam and tooth cleaning. Regular visits to the dentist will help prevent tooth loss and gum disease. (For more information about dental care, see pp. 242-251.)

#7: Build a Partnership with Your Physician

TODAY people are taking a more active role in their health care. That's a good thing. After all, each of us is the person most responsible for our own state of health. One key to being an active health care consumer is building a strong partnership with your main, or primary, physician. You and your doctor need to work together to make the best possible decisions about your health care.

You want your doctor to be well qualified, of course, and someone you can trust. You need to be able to talk openly with your doctor about your personal concerns. And your doctor should provide you with clear, thorough information in return.

Why You Need a Primary Care Physician

It's important to have one doctor who knows you and your health history well. Such a doctor is called a *primary care physician*—a nonspecialty doctor who provides general medical care. The most common types of primary care physicians used by older adults are *family practice physicians* (specializing in the general care of people of all ages), *internists* (specializing in the care of adults), and *geriatricians* (specializing in the care of older adults).

Your primary care physician is the doctor you go to for your regular checkups and preventive exams. If you need to see a specialist, your primary care physician will refer you to one.

Having a primary care physician has many advantages. He or she will have your complete medical file, for example, and know your entire medical history. That will reduce the chance that you'll have to repeat a medical procedure or test unnecessarily. (Make sure all your past medical records, reports, and tests are sent to your primary care physician.)

Yet there's an even bigger advantage in having a primary care physician: With such a doctor you can build a long-term, trusting relationship.

How to Find a Primary Care Physician

You may already have a primary care physician you know and trust. But if you do not (if you have recently moved to a new city, for example, or if your doctor has retired), here are three steps you can take to find a new one:

1. Make a list of names of doctor "candidates." Ask friends and family members for recommendations of doctors they like and trust. If you belong to a managed care plan, call their customer service line. Ask for the names of primary care physicians located near you who are affiliated with the plan. You can also call your local medical association for names of primary care physicians in your area.

2. Narrow your list down to two or three names, then call the office of each doctor. Tell the doctor's staff that you are looking for a primary care physician. Ask if the doctor is taking new patients, accepts Medicare patients, makes house calls, and so on. (For a list of questions to ask the staff, see p. 46.) Note how the staff treats you. It could reflect the attitude of the doctor.

3. Interview the doctor. It's best to do this interview in person. Be aware that some doctors will charge you for this interview. Tell the office staff of your intent to interview the doctor when you schedule the appointment. Ask them up front what that fee will be. Take a list of prepared questions with you (see p. 46). Pay attention to how the doctor answers your questions. Does he or she explain things in terms you understand? Do you feel comfortable enough with the doctor to share personal information? Does the doctor listen well to your concerns?

Don't wait until you have an emergency or a major health problem to find a primary care physician. Start looking now. You may need time to find just the right doctor. And remember: It's all right to be choosy. After all, it's *your* health.

How to Prepare for Visits to Your Physician

Before leaving for your physician's office, take some time to prepare for the visit. This will make it more likely that you'll leave the appointment well informed and satisfied with the care you received.

Here are some things you can do to prepare:

- Make a list of what you want to discuss. Write down questions that you want to ask during the visit.

PHYSICIANS AND THEIR SPECIALTIES

Physician	Specialty
Allergist	Allergies and other conditions affecting the immune system
Anesthesiologist	The use of anesthetics for safe and painless surgery
Cardiologist	Diseases of the heart
Dermatologist	Diseases and conditions of the skin
Emergency medicine specialist	Emergency care of the severely ill or injured
Endocrinologist	Disorders of the hormonal system
Family physician	Medical care of all family members
Gastroenterologist	Disorders of the stomach, esophagus, pancreas, intestines, liver, and gallbladder
Geriatrician	Medical care of older adults
Gynecologist	Disorders of the female reproductive system
Internist	Medical care of adults of all ages
Nephrologist	Diseases and problems of the kidneys
Neurologist	Disorders of the nervous system
Ophthalmologist	Diseases and problems of the eyes
Orthopedist	Problems involving the skeleton and joints
Otolaryngologist	Conditions of the ear, nose, and throat
Physiatrist	Treatment of muscle and bone disorders
Podiatrist	Conditions of the feet
Preventive medicine physician	Disease prevention and occupational medicine
Psychiatrist	Treatment of mental and emotional illnesses
Radiologist	The use of X-ray and other imaging techniques for diagnosis and treatment
Urologist	Diseases of the urinary tract

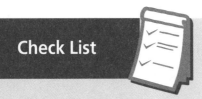

Check List

QUESTIONS TO ASK WHEN CHOOSING A PHYSICIAN

Ask these questions of the physician's office staff:

☑ Is the physician covered by your health insurance plan?

☑ Does the physician accept Medicare?

☑ What hospital does the physician admit patients to? Is the hospital covered by your insurance plan?

☑ What days/hours does the physician see patients?

☑ Does the physician ever make house calls?

☑ How far in advance do you have to make a routine appointment? An urgent appointment?

☑ What is the length of an average visit?

☑ In case of an emergency, how fast can you see the physician?

☑ Who takes care of patients after hours or when the physician is away?

Ask these questions directly of the physician:

☑ Does the physician have many older patients? What are his or her views on health and aging? Does the physician treat illnesses in an older person aggressively, or does he or she view illness as "a natural part of aging"?

☑ How does the physician feel about involving a patient's family in care decisions?

☑ Will the physician honor living wills, durable powers of attorney for health care, and other advance directives?

☑ Does the physician work with patients when they go into adult day care or move to a nursing home?

- If you're having symptoms you want to discuss with your physician, jot down as much information about them as you can. For example, write down what the symptoms are, when they started, what they feel like, what triggers them, and what relieves them (such as resting or taking a medication).

- Make a list of all the medications you're taking. Be sure to include over-the-counter drugs, vitamins, and other supplements (including herbal). If you prefer, you can take your medications in their original containers to the appointment.

- Take along any information your physician may need, including insurance cards, names of your other doctors (including alternative practitioners, such as acupuncturists and massage therapists), and your medical records.

- If you use glasses or hearing aids, take them with you to the appointment. Also, let your physician and his or her staff know if you have difficulty seeing or hearing.

- Consider bringing a family member or friend. It may be helpful to have someone else with you. This person can help you remember the questions you wanted to ask and what the physician told you.

What to Do During the Visit

- Listen carefully to what your physician tells you. Ask questions if you don't understand something.

- Take notes. Write down the information and instructions your physician gives you. Or (with your physician's permission) bring along a tape recorder.

- Ask your physician if he or she has any prepared information, such as brochures, cassette tapes, or videotapes, about your health condition or treatment that you can take home with you. If your physician does not have this information, he or she may be able to recommend other sources that do.

- Be honest with your physician. Don't withhold any information about your eating or exercising habits, your smoking history, any history of alcohol or substance abuse, supplements you take (including herbal), and other care you receive. If you're seeing an alternative practitioner, let your physician know. Your physician needs truthful information if he or she is to give you the best care possible.

- Stick to the point. Doing so will make the best use of your time.

- Share your point of view. Your physician may not realize that you don't understand something or that you are feeling rushed. Tell your physician when you want more information. Your physician may be able to set aside more time for you. Or the two of you may be able to arrange to have a phone conversation in the near future.

What You Should Expect from Your Doctor

As part of the doctor-patient relationship, it is important that a doctor communicate well with patients. Your doctor should

- explain things so that you understand them. This includes information about your condition, any tests you need, and any procedures you may undergo.

- take the time to answer your questions thoroughly and make sure that you are satisfied with the answers.

- give you specific instructions for treating your condition and taking any medications that are prescribed. He or she should also tell you when you should return for a follow-up visit, if necessary.

- return your phone calls in a reasonable amount of time.

- treat you with respect.

- know about the latest advances in medicine and be able to answer your questions about them.

Source: American Medical Association

Questions to Ask Your Doctor Before Having Surgery

Most of the millions of medical operations performed each year are not emergencies. They are elective surgeries—in other words, a physician has recommended the surgery to a patient. The patient can then decide whether to have the surgery and, if so, when and where.

If you are facing elective surgery, you should ask your physician and your surgeon the following questions. The answers they give will help you make the best decision about your surgery. Be sure to ask the doctors to explain their answers clearly and thoroughly.

1. What operation are you recommending?

2. Why do I need the operation?

3. Are there alternatives to surgery? What conservative measures could we try first?

4. What are the benefits of having the operation?

5. What are the risks of having the operation?

6. What if I don't have this operation?

7. Where can I get a second opinion?

8. How many times have you done this operation? How did the patients do?

9. Where will the operation be done?

10. What kind of anesthesia will I need?

11. How long will it take me to recover?

12. How much will the operation cost? Who pays these costs?

13. How will the operation affect my quality of life?

How to Choose a Hospital

Not all hospitals are alike. One hospital may be better staffed and equipped than another to do a particular procedure. A hospital that does many successful coronary bypass surgeries, for example, may not be the best hospital to go to for **cancer** treatment. Each hospital has its own advantages and special characteristics.

Your physician can help you choose the hospital that is best suited for your needs. But you should also do some research on your own.

• Check to see if the hospital is accredited by a nationally recognized accrediting organization, such as the Joint Commission on Accreditation of Healthcare Organizations (JCAHO).

• Find out how often the specific procedure you need is done at the hospital. What is the hospital's success rate in carrying out the procedure?

• Visit the hospital. Does it appear clean? Are the patient rooms comfortable? Will you have privacy in your room? Do you feel the hospital is a place where you will be treated with dignity and respect?

• Find out how the hospital plans to keep your physician and other members of your health team informed about your progress during recuperation. Also, how will you or your family be kept up-to-date on your progress?

- Does the hospital have social workers to help patients and their families access emotional, financial, and physical support services?

- Ask the hospital for a written description of its services and fees. Will the hospital provide financial assistance if you need it?

- Find out what kind of care the hospital provides after you leave its facility. Will the hospital send a nurse to your home for a post-operation checkup? What kind of training will the hospital give you and your family to make sure you continue your care in your home?

- Request a copy of the hospital's patient rights and responsibilities form. Also, ask about the hospital's policies concerning confidentiality of medical records.

#8: Stay Connected

As you age it's important that you stay connected with other people. Studies have shown that people who remain socially active live longer, healthier, and happier lives. Not only do they have fewer health problems, they are also less likely to suffer from **depression**.

Even if you live alone, you needn't be lonely. There are plenty of ways you can become involved in your community. Here are a few ideas:

Join (or Start) a Social Group

Most communities have a wide variety of social clubs or organizations that people of all ages can join. These can range from backyard gardening clubs to groups that regularly travel to foreign lands. To find these groups, try calling your local chamber of commerce. Churches, synagogues, and other places of worship also have groups that organize social events for visitors as well as members.

A good place to socialize with other older adults is through your local senior center. Most offer lunches, classes, organized outings, dances, and other functions. You can also organize your own social group. Call some friends and start a monthly book or craft group, for example. Or arrange to go with friends on regular outings to theater or sports events.

If transportation is a problem, ask your senior center or local transit system about special senior transportation programs.

Volunteer

Volunteering is a great way to put your skills and life experience to work for your community. It is also a great way of meeting new people and making friends. The types of volunteer opportunities that are available to older adults are almost endless. You can help teach children to read, feed meals to the poor, offer comfort to a hospital patient, lead museum tours, build a house for a needy family, and much, much more.

Your local senior center should have information about volunteer opportunities in your area. Or you could call a local institution, such as a hospital or school, and ask how you could help. You could also join a national service organization for older adults, such as RSVP (Retired Senior Volunteer Program), Volunteers in Parks, or the Service Corps of Retired Executives (SCORE). All of these organizations are part of the National Senior Service Corps (Senior Corps), a network of volunteer programs for people aged 55 and over. The Senior Corps can connect you to many local organizations that need your help. (For information about how to reach the Senior Corps, see the "Resources" section of this book.)

Take a Class

Taking a class is a great way of meeting people who share the same interest as you. You could take a class in something practical, like stock investing or home repair, or in something more creative, like memoir writing or opera appreciation. Many schools, colleges, and universities offer these "continuing education" classes to people of all ages. The classes are usually reasonably priced and frequently offer discounts to older adults. Some universities have "elder institutes" geared specially to the interests of older adults. Call your local educational institutions and ask for a catalog of their continuing education classes.

Many hospitals offer classes and support groups for people with chronic illnesses such as **diabetes**, **coronary heart disease**, or **Parkinson's disease**. They also offer preventive classes—how to cook heart-healthy meals, for example, or how to reduce stress. Call your local hospital for more information.

Finally, you may want to consider returning to a college or university to pursue a degree. Older adults of all ages (even some in their 80s and 90s!) are going back to college in record numbers.

Reach for Religion

Attending church, synagogue, or another religious institution regularly may lengthen your life. That's what a National Institute on Aging study found. Even after taking in such factors as smoking, age, and chronic health conditions, older Americans who attended religious meetings each week lived 28 percent longer than those who stayed at home, according to the study.

The researchers think that the social support offered by religious institutions may help keep the immune system strong. Indeed, other studies have linked religious attendance to lower blood pressure, fewer cases of **stroke**, less **depression**, and better compliance with taking medications.

Many religious institutions offer a variety of special support groups and services (including transportation to events) to their older visitors and members. If you do not already belong to a religious institution, you can find one near you by looking in the Yellow Pages of your local phone book.

Stay Physically Active

The more you exercise your body, the more energy you'll have to pursue social activities. But exercising can also be a great way of becoming socially involved with others. You can sign up for an exercise class at your local YWCA or YMCA, for example. Many communities also offer exercise classes at high schools, community park buildings, hospitals, and senior centers. Some classes are specially designed for people with a chronic illness or disability, such as **arthritis**.

You could also form your own exercise group. For example, you could arrange to meet some friends at your local mall for regular walking sessions. Another option is joining a sports league just for older people. Many sports have such leagues, including running, bowling, tennis, golf, and swimming. For information about leagues in your area, contact your local senior center.

Major Health Concerns

There's no getting around it: Age is a risk factor for many major illnesses, from **Alzheimer's disease** to **stroke**. The longer we live, the greater the likelihood that we'll experience a major illness.

That's the bad news. Now here's the good news: Age is never the *only* cause of an illness. It's just one of many risk factors. Genetics can also play a role. Some illnesses seem to run in families. But by far the biggest risk factor for most major illnesses is lifestyle habits—what you eat, how often you exercise, whether you see your physician regularly, and so on.

If you take care of yourself—by following, for example, the prescription for health outlined on pp. 1-53—you may be able to avoid the major illnesses and conditions often associated with getting older. Or, at the very least, you may be able to slow down the onset or the progress of these illnesses.

The major health concerns listed on the following pages are all chronic, or long-term, diseases. Once you develop a chronic illness, you must usually live with it for the rest of your life. That can be difficult, sometimes even devastating. But it *is* possible to live an active, productive life with a chronic illness. Millions of people do it every day.

If you have a chronic illness, you can enhance the quality of your life by

- learning about your illness;
- becoming an active participant in your care; and
- finding out about resources and support in your community.

You can start by reading about your particular illness on the following pages.

Caring for Someone with a Major Illness

IF you are providing care to a relative or friend with a major, long-term illness, you are not alone. It is estimated that about 25 million Americans are "family caregivers"—people who out of love, concern, or a simple sense of duty are assisting a chronically ill or disabled person with day-to-day tasks. The vast majority of older adults with chronic illnesses—about 80 percent—are cared for by family members. Family caregivers find, manage, or provide a wide range of necessary assistance. They help with housekeeping, finances, meals, bathing, dressing, shopping, transportation, and more. They also provide love and emotional support.

Caring for a person with a major or chronic illness can be a satisfying and meaningful experience. But it can also be stressful—emotionally, financially, spiritually, and physically. It's not unusual for family caregivers to become depressed or anxious or to develop physical ailments.

If you are caring for a loved one with a chronic illness, it's important that you find practical ways to cope. The most common mistake family caregivers make is not taking care of themselves. You need to schedule regular breaks from your caregiving responsibilities. That will require developing a network of support from both family and outside sources. Fortunately there are many organizations that can help you develop that support network. You'll find some of them listed in the "Resources" section of this book.

10 Tips for Family Caregivers

1. Choose to take charge of your life, and don't let your loved one's illness or disability always take center stage.

2. Remember to be good to yourself. Love, honor, and value yourself. You're doing a very hard job, and you deserve some quality time just for you.

3. Watch out for signs of **depression**, and don't delay in getting professional help when you need it.

4. When people offer to help, accept the offer and suggest specific things that they can do.

5. Educate yourself about your loved one's condition. Information is empowering.

6. There's a difference between caring and doing. Be open to technologies and ideas that promote your loved one's independence.

7. Trust your instincts. Most of the time they'll lead you in the right direction.

8. Grieve for your losses, and then allow yourself to dream new dreams.

9. Stand up for your rights as a caregiver and a citizen.

10. Seek support from other caregivers. There is great strength in knowing you are not alone.

Source: National Family Caregivers Association

Self-Test

Do You Have Caregiver Burnout?

Are you not eating properly?
❏ Yes   ❏ No

Are you becoming more emotional?
❏ Yes   ❏ No

Are you feeling overwhelmed?
❏ Yes   ❏ No

Are you starting to withdraw from social activities you used to enjoy?
❏ Yes   ❏ No

Are you seeing friends and family members less often?
❏ Yes   ❏ No

Are you having trouble focusing on work or other activities?
❏ Yes   ❏ No

Are you taking less care with your personal appearance?
❏ Yes   ❏ No

If you answered "Yes" to any of these questions, you may be experiencing caregiver burnout. Ask for help. Sources may include family, friends, church members, home health agencies, social service departments, and other community services.

CAREGIVER'S BILL OF RIGHTS

I have the right...

- to take care of myself. This is not an act of selfishness. It will give me the capability of taking better care of my relative.

- to seek help from others, even though my relatives may object. I recognize the limits of my own endurance and strength.

- to maintain facets of my own life that do not include the person I care for, just as I would if he or she were healthy. I know that I do everything that I reasonably can for this person, and I have the right to do some things just for myself.

- to get angry, be depressed, and express other difficult feelings occasionally.

- to reject any attempts by my relative (either conscious or unconscious) to manipulate me through guilt and/or **depression**.

- to receive consideration, affection, forgiveness, and acceptance from my loved one for what I do, for as long as I offer these qualities in return.

- to take pride in what I am accomplishing and to applaud the courage it has sometimes taken to meet the needs of my relative.

- to protect my individuality and my right to make a life for myself that will sustain me in the time when my relative no longer needs my full-time help.

- to expect and demand that as new strides are made in finding resources to aid physically and mentally impaired persons in our country, similar strides will be made toward aiding and supporting caregivers.

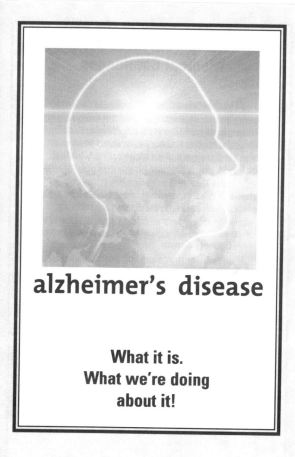

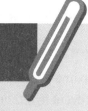

...tive condition in which brain cells break ... loss and changes in behavior and ...he affected person eventually becomes ...spects of daily life.

...after age 65. People with the disease live an ...appear. Some people, however, live with the ...imer's disease gets worse over time. As yet ...e research in the field.

...arily strikes people over age 65, it is not a ...6 percent of older people have Alzheimer's

...believe that more than one factor is involved in triggering the disease.

Treatment

Nothing can stop or reverse Alzheimer's disease. But there are medications that may help slow its progression. Other medications can

Symptoms

- Dramatic changes in mood or behavior; may include depression or suspiciousness

- Increased tendency to misplace things

- Confusion, disorientation

- Loss of interest in usual pursuits

- Problems with tasks that require abstract thinking

When to Seek Help

- If you notice increasingly frequent or severe memory lapses in yourself or an older family member or loved one

  ▶ *Call your nurse information service or physician.*

- If you notice persistent and unexplained personality or behavioral changes in yourself or an older family member or loved one

  ▶ *Call your nurse information service or physician.*

Important: A person who is experiencing symptoms of Alzheimer's disease may not be aware of having these problems. A family member or friend may need to take the initiative to seek medical help.

help with some of the mood and behavioral changes associated with the disease, such as **depression**, sleeplessness, and delusions.

Prevention

No one knows what causes Alzheimer's disease. So no one knows for sure what can prevent it, either. Some studies have suggested, however, that several therapies may have potential to prevent or slow the progression of the disease. These therapies include nonsteroidal anti-inflammatory drugs (NSAIDs) such as ibuprofen and naproxen; estrogen supplements; vitamin E; Selegiline (a prescription drug used to treat **Parkinson's disease**); and ginkgo biloba, a Chinese herb. More research is needed, however, to establish if these therapies have any real value.

Caution: Each of these therapies has potential side effects that may be harmful to your health. Talk to your physician before taking any of them.

If You Are Taking Care of Someone with Alzheimer's

- Try to keep your loved one's living environment as stable and routine as possible. When you are away, leave written reminders and directions to help your loved one do simple everyday tasks.

- People with Alzheimer's disease sometimes wander off and become lost. Make sure your loved one has an ID bracelet or card that tells whom to call in an emergency.

- Many people with Alzheimer's have trouble sleeping at night. To help your loved one sleep better, try keeping him or her more active during the day. Discourage afternoon napping. Also limit caffeine and sweets to the morning hours.

- Exercise can sometimes help a person with Alzheimer's talk more. Studies suggest that walking activates areas of the brain linked to speech. Encourage your loved one to go for a daily walk with you.

- Get help for yourself. Caring for someone with Alzheimer's can be very stressful. More than 80 percent of Alzheimer's caregivers report that they often feel high levels of stress. More than half say they suffer from **depression**. Many caregivers are often unaware that they are under stress. Others simply don't know where to turn for help. Fortunately many good resources are available for Alzheimer's caregivers. The organizations listed in the "Resources" section of this book are a good place to start.

> ### What is...?
>
> **...dementia?** It is a general term meaning loss of brain function. Symptoms include loss of memory, mental confusion, personality changes, and inability to function in daily life. Other symptoms may include **depression**, **anxiety**, or suspiciousness. Alzheimer's disease is the most common cause of dementia. But dementia has other causes as well, including repeated **stroke**; chronic abuse of alcohol; head injuries; and certain illnesses, such as **AIDS**.

How Will Having Alzheimer's Disease Change My Life?

Living with Alzheimer's is a different experience for each person with the disease. In some people the disease progresses quickly. In other people it develops slowly, over many years. But you should expect to experience many changes.

As the disease progresses, you will find it increasingly difficult to think and remember, learn new information, and make decisions. Things that were once familiar may become unfamiliar. You may find yourself getting lost. Understanding what other people are saying to you—and getting them to understand your words—may also become a problem.

Eventually you will need help with your day-to-day care. It's best if you and your family start making plans for this care soon after your diagnosis. For help in doing this, contact the Alzheimer's Association, which is listed in the "Resources" section of this book. They can provide you and your family with information and support.

Discovering you have Alzheimer's can be an emotionally devastating experience. Living with the illness can lead to frustration, anger, and **depression**. You may benefit from talking with a psychologist or other qualified counselor about your concerns. Ask your physician for referrals.

Arthritis

Arthritis is a general term for a group of disorders that can cause pain, stiffness, and swelling in the joints. Any joint can be affected, including the knees, hips, and fingers. Arthritis is usually chronic. It is common among older adults, affecting about half of all people aged 65 and older.

More than 100 types of arthritis have been identified. Many have different symptoms and treatments. The three most common kinds of arthritis in older people are osteoarthritis, rheumatoid arthritis, and gout.

Symptoms

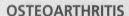

OSTEOARTHRITIS

- Pain or stiffness in or near a joint; movement usually makes the pain worse
- Bony swelling in a joint
- Crackling noises when you move a joint
- Inflammation (swelling, redness, and tenderness) in a joint

RHEUMATOID ARTHRITIS

- Tender, warm, red, swollen joints
- Fatigue, occasional low fever, loss of appetite—a general feeling of being unwell
- Morning stiffness and pain that lasts 30 minutes or longer
- Dry eyes and mouth

GOUT

- Sudden, intense pain in a joint, often the wrist, big toe, or knee
- Redness, swelling around affected joint
- Low fever

When to Seek Help

• If you suddenly develop a red, swollen joint	▶ *Call your physician now.*
• If any of the symptoms of **arthritis** (p. 63) last longer than two weeks	▶ *Call your nurse information service or physician.*

- *Osteoarthritis*, once known as *degenerative joint disease*, is the most common type of arthritis in older people. It happens when the protective layer of cartilage between bones wears away. The exposed bones rub together. The rubbing sometimes causes rough spots, known as *spurs*, to develop. The result: damaged muscles and nerves, which can cause pain and stiffness. Osteoarthritis usually affects the joints of the hands, knees, and hips.

- *Rheumatoid arthritis*, sometimes called *rheumatism*, occurs when the membrane that surrounds a joint becomes inflamed and thickened. This causes pain and stiffness, especially on awakening in the morning. Rheumatoid arthritis most often affects the joints of the hands, but those of the arms, legs, and feet can also become inflamed. This type of arthritis can also damage other parts of the body, including the eyes, lungs, and heart.

- *Gout* is caused when blood levels of uric acid—one of the body's waste products—get too high. The excess uric acid forms crystals in the spaces around joints. The body's immune system attacks these crystals, causing the joint to become inflamed and painful. Gout affects the toes, ankles, elbows, wrists, and hands. Gout attacks are usually quite sudden and very painful. About 90 percent of gout sufferers are older men.

Causes

Osteoarthritis is not an inevitable part of aging. But it can result from old injuries or overuse of joints. Being overweight, which puts stress on knee joints, can also increase the risk. Osteoarthritis also tends to run in families.

Rheumatoid arthritis is believed to be an *autoimmune disease*—a disease in which the body mistakenly attacks its own tissue. Scientists are not sure why the body attacks the membrane around joints.

Gout can be triggered by many factors. Drinking too much alcohol and eating a diet rich in foods that raise uric acid levels (organ meats, broths, gravies, sardines, anchovies, and sweetbreads) may lead to a gout attack in susceptible people. Other factors include surgery, a sudden and severe illness, kidney failure, certain medications, chemotherapy, and long-term use of aspirin.

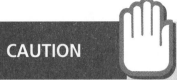

CAUTION

Beware of unproven "cures" for arthritis. Some, such as wearing copper bracelets, are harmless, but also useless. Others, such as ingesting snake venom or taking high doses of vitamins, can be dangerous. Don't risk your health—or waste your money—on unproven cures. Talk to your physician first.

Treatment

Osteoarthritis and rheumatoid arthritis cannot be cured. But treating the arthritis can help reduce pain and swelling and keep joints from becoming damaged further. Treatments include medications, special exercises, use of heat or cold, and weight control. In more severe cases surgery may also be recommended to smooth rough joint surfaces or replace a damaged joint.

Gout can be treated with medications that reduce uric acid in the blood. Your physician may also advise you to stop using alcohol, lose weight, and avoid trigger foods.

Living with Arthritis

- Exercise daily. Moving your joints will help reduce pain and strengthen the muscles around the joints.

- Take rest breaks during the day. Give your joints time to recover between periods of activity.

- Apply heat or cold to sore joints. Heat relaxes your muscles and stimulates circulation. Try warm towels, hot packs, a bath, or a shower. Or take a swim in a heated pool. Cold numbs sore joints and reduces inflammation and swelling. A bag of ice or frozen vegetables wrapped in a towel can be used as a cold pack. Make sure your skin is dry and healthy before applying heat or cold to your body. Don't use this treatment for more than 15 to 20 minutes at a time. Also, don't use cold packs if you have a circulatory disorder.

- Learn relaxation techniques. Such techniques can help you release tension in your muscles, which in turn will help reduce pain. The Arthritis Foundation (see p. 342) has a self-help course that includes relaxation therapy.

- Consider massage. Soft-tissue massage can help control pain and increase the motion of your joints. Ask your physician for a referral to a professional who is knowledgeable and has had experience giving massages to people with arthritis.

- Consider other treatments. Some people with arthritis get pain relief from biofeedback, acupuncture, or a TENS (transcutaneous electrical nerve stimulator). *Biofeedback* uses electrical equipment to teach you how to control your body's physical reaction to stress and pain. *Acupuncture* is an ancient Chinese method of pain control; small needles are inserted into specific points of the body to block pain. A *TENS* is a small device that blocks pain by sending a mild electrical current to nerves in the affected area of the body. You wear the device during the day and turn it off and on as needed. If you want to try any of these treatments, ask your physician for a referral to a trained professional. Check with your health plan about coverage.

- Join an arthritis support group. Sharing your feelings and frustrations about your arthritis with others can make living with this chronic disease easier. A support group can help you realize that you are not alone, and it can provide you with many helpful ideas and resources. Your physician or your local chapter of the Arthritis Foundation can help you find a support group near you.

How Will Having Arthritis Change My Life?

Your arthritis will require you to make changes in your daily routine. To keep the disease under control, you will need to schedule times each day to exercise and rest, even when you are feeling well. Arthritis can cause great fatigue. You will need to learn how to pace your activities throughout the day.

Arthritis is a chronic illness, but its symptoms can come and go. You may feel good one day and miserable the next. The pain can change even from hour to hour. On some days you may find it difficult to do even routine tasks such as cooking and cleaning. On other days you may feel pain-free and have a great deal of energy.

Your family and friends may not understand the on-and-off nature of arthritis. They may accuse you of exaggerating your symptoms. You may find such attitudes difficult to deal with. You may choose to ignore such comments, or you may want to use the situation to educate others about arthritis and its symptoms. For help in doing this, contact the Arthritis Foundation, which is listed in the "Resources" section of this book. They can provide you with information and support.

Having arthritis is a challenge. It can affect your self-image and lead to frustration, anger, and **depression**. Adjusting to living with the disease takes time and patience. You may benefit from talking with a psychologist or other qualified counselor about your concerns. Ask your physician for referrals.

Cancer

CANCER starts when a healthy cell mutates, or changes, and then multiplies in an uncontrolled way. The abnormal cells keep dividing. They cluster together, forming a tumor. The tumor damages surrounding healthy cells, robbing them of their nutrients and oxygen. Cancerous tumor cells may eventually enter the bloodstream or lymph system. They can then spread to other parts of the body—a process called *metastasis*.

Although most cancers form tumors, not all tumors are *cancerous*, or malignant. Some tumors are *self-contained*, or benign. These tumors may stop growing and don't travel to other sites in the body. They are rarely life-threatening.

According to the American Cancer Society, about half of all men and one-third of all women will develop cancer during their lifetimes. A cancer diagnosis once meant almost certain death. But today millions of people are living with cancer or have been cured of the disease.

Causes

One-third of all cancer deaths in the United States is caused by cigarette smoking. Another third is linked to the foods we do—or don't—eat. Consuming too much alcohol, fat, and foods that have been smoked, cured, pickled, or charred is a risk factor. So is eating too few fruits, vegetables, and whole grains—foods rich in antioxidants and fiber, which may reduce the risk for cancer.

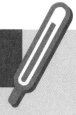

Symptoms

- Change in bowel or bladder habits

- A sore that does not heal

- Unusual bleeding or discharge

- Thickening or lump in the breast or elsewhere

- Chronic **indigestion** or difficulty swallowing

- Obvious change in a wart, mole, or mouth sore

- Persistent cough or hoarseness

Other risk factors include too much exposure to sunlight, radiation, and cancer-causing chemicals such as asbestos, vinyl chloride, and arsenic. Research also suggests that certain types of cancer run in families.

Treatment

The standard treatments for cancer are surgery, chemotherapy, and/or radiation therapy. Surgery involves removing all or part of a cancerous tumor, and sometimes surrounding healthy tissue. Chemo-therapy treats the cancer with special drugs that destroy cancer cells. It is most often given *intravenously* (through a needle inserted into a vein). Radiation therapy uses high-energy X-rays or rays from radioactive substances to destroy tumors.

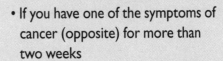

When to Seek Help

- If you have one of the symptoms of cancer (opposite) for more than two weeks

▼

Call your nurse information service or physician.

Chemotherapy and radiation therapies may affect healthy as well as cancerous cells. As a result, they often cause unwanted side effects. Chemotherapy side effects can include nausea, vomiting, mouth sores, and temporary hair loss. Radiation may also cause these side effects, depending on the area of the body being treated. Your physician can give you medications and other therapies that can help lessen some of the side effects. Most side effects disappear when the treatment ends.

Some cancers, such as those of the breast and prostate, are now sometimes treated with hormones. Other new treatments include biological therapies that use the body's immune system, either directly or indirectly, to fight cancer or to lessen side effects that may be caused by some cancer treatments.

Early Detection

Improvements in treatment over the past two decades have made it possible for greater numbers of people with cancer to live longer and healthier lives. But the key to successful cancer treatment is early detection. If cancerous cells can be destroyed before they have spread, a person with cancer has a greater chance for survival. So be sure to schedule preventive checkups and cancer screenings with your physician.

Common Cancers

Lung, colorectal, breast, and prostate cancers are the four most common cancers in the United States. Lung and colorectal cancer are discussed here. You'll find information about breast and other women's cancers on pp. 220-227 and about prostate and testicular cancers—"men's" cancers—on pp. 234-239. For a discussion of oral cancer see p. 256.

Lung Cancer

Lung cancer is the leading cause of cancer death in the United States. It's also one of the most preventable types of cancer. Almost all—90 percent—of lung cancer is caused by smoking. If you smoke a pack of cigarettes a day, you are 20 times more likely than a nonsmoker to develop lung cancer.

Lung cancer usually strikes people over the age of 50. That's because the disease can take many years to develop. Symptoms include the following:

- a persistent cough or hoarseness
- chest pain
- weight loss and loss of appetite
- shortness of breath
- recurring infections, such as bronchitis and **pneumonia**

If you have any of these symptoms, you should call your physician right away. And if you smoke, stop. (For tips on how to quit smoking, see pp. 30-31.)

Colorectal Cancer

Colorectal cancer—cancer of the large intestine, the colon, and rectum—is the second leading cancer killer in the United States. Just being over the age of 50 puts you at risk for colorectal cancer. So does eating a high-fat, low-fiber diet. Other risk factors include having *polyps* (noncancerous growths on the inner wall of the large intestine) or *ulcerative colitis* (an inflammation of the lining of the colon). People with a family history of colorectal cancer are also at higher risk.

Colorectal cancer is very curable if caught early. So it's important to know its major symptoms:

- diarrhea or other change in bowel habits lasting 10 days or more

- blood in the stool

- unexplained anemia

- abdominal discomfort or pain

- weight loss

It's also important that everyone over the age of 50 be screened regularly for colorectal cancer. Each year you should get a *fecal occult blood test*, a test used to check for hidden blood in the stool. Every three to five years you should have a *sigmoidoscopy*, an exam that uses a lighted instrument to examine the rectum and lower colon. Your physician may also recommend other screening tests.

Did You Know?

People who drink more than four cups of green tea daily have a lower overall risk of cancer. Researchers believe green tea may have an anticancer compound.

You can take many steps to prevent colorectal cancer. These include the following:

- Eat plenty of fresh fruits, vegetables, and whole grains.

- Cut back on meat and other high-fat foods.

- Exercise daily.

- Talk to your physician about taking aspirin daily. Some studies have shown that aspirin may help prevent colorectal cancer.

Prevention

- Do not smoke or use chewing tobacco.

- Stay out of the sun, especially during peak hours (10 A.M. to 3 P.M.). When outdoors, wear protective clothing and use sunscreen to protect your skin from ultraviolet rays.

- Eat most of your foods from plant sources—fruits, vegetables, and whole grains.

- Limit the amount of high-fat foods in your diet, particularly from animal sources.

- Exercise regularly.

- Maintain a healthy weight.

- Drink alcohol in moderation, if at all.

- Get regular screenings for cancer (see p. 41).

Did You Know?

The radioactive gas radon is the second leading cause of lung cancer. Radon is found naturally in soil and rocks. It can seep into homes and other buildings. The Environmental Protection Agency (EPA) estimates that nearly 1 out of every 15 homes in the United States has indoor radon levels at or above the recommended limit. The EPA and many health organizations recommend that people get their homes tested for radon. For information on how to do this, call your local health department.

How Will Having Cancer Change My Life?

Each person lives with cancer in a different way. After the diagnosis you may experience shock, fear, and even **depression**. The important thing to remember is that with today's research advances, many cancers are curable. Talking with your physician, friends, and family can help you work through your feelings. Try to seek out people who have a positive attitude. You may also benefit from talking with a psychologist or other qualified counselor about your concerns. Ask your physician for referrals.

Some cancer treatments can make you feel very ill. You may find it difficult, if not impossible, to continue with your usual activities. Treatment may also make you feel uncomfortable about your body. You may feel unattractive sexually. It's important to discuss these feelings openly with your partner.

Cancer can be lonely. But you don't have to deal with it alone. Fortunately many organizations offer support to people with this disease. Ask your physician for referrals, or contact the organizations listed in the "Resources" section of this book.

Chronic Obstructive Pulmonary Disease (COPD)

TWO lung diseases—chronic bronchitis and emphysema—often occur together. That's why physicians refer to these diseases under the general term "chronic obstructive pulmonary disease," or COPD for short.

- *Chronic bronchitis* is a disease that affects the bronchial passages that carry air to and from the lungs. The passages become swollen and clogged with extra mucus. The result: coughing and shortness of breath.

- *Emphysema* is a disease that destroys the walls of the air sacs, or *alveoli*, deep within the lungs. Breathing, especially exhaling, becomes very difficult.

Causes

Smoking is the cause of about 80 to 90 percent of COPD cases. Frequent lung infections and exposure to certain industrial pollutants can also bring on the disease. Some people are born with a rare form of emphysema that shows up when they reach their 30s or 40s.

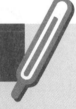

Symptoms

- Chronic cough that may or may not produce phlegm
- Frequent clearing of the throat
- Chronic shortness of breath

Treatment

No treatment can make your lungs healthy again. But you can do things to keep the disease from getting worse. First, stop smoking. It's also important to take steps to protect yourself against **colds and flu**. With COPD your body is less able to fight off these kinds of infections.

If you have COPD, you should see your physician regularly. COPD can be life-threatening, and it's important that it be monitored closely. Your physician will show

When to Seek Help

- If you have been diagnosed with COPD and your complexion turns blue or purple

  ▶ *Seek emergency care immediately.*

- If you have a chronic cough that does not go away after several weeks

  ▶ *Call your physician now.*

- If you often become breathless after doing a simple activity, such as climbing a flight of stairs

  ▶ *Call your physician.*

- If you have been diagnosed with COPD and develop gradual swelling in the legs or ankles

  ▶ *Call your nurse information service or physician.*

- If you have been diagnosed with COPD and experience shortness of breath when you are resting or doing minimal physical exercise

  ▶ *Call your nurse information service or physician.*

- If you have been diagnosed with COPD and are coughing up phlegm that is thicker than usual or that has blood in it

  ▶ *Call your nurse information service or physician.*

you how to do breathing exercises. He or she will also teach you how to cough in a controlled way to remove extra mucus from your lungs. Other treatments for COPD include bronchodilators, which open up air passages in the lungs; antibiotics, which help fight bacterial infections; and exercise, which helps strengthen the lungs.

Some people with COPD need at-home oxygen therapy. Surgery is also sometimes an option. The treatments that are right for you will depend on how severe your disease is.

Living with COPD

- Stop smoking. If you don't stop smoking, your illness will almost certainly worsen.

- Avoid secondhand smoke, dust, and other air pollutants.

- Take daily walks. Exercise is important for people with COPD, and walking is a great way to get that exercise. Be sure to avoid highly polluted areas.

- Eat healthful foods. Eating well can help protect you against infection.

- Maintain your ideal weight. Being overweight can make it harder to take a full breath. In addition, having COPD increases your risk for developing **coronary heart disease**, and being overweight can put added strain on your heart.

- Get vaccinated against influenza and pneumococcal **pneumonia**.

- Avoid exposure to **colds and flu**. See your doctor or follow your doctor's instructions at the beginning of any respiratory infection.

How Will Having Chronic Obstructive Pulmonary Disease Change My Life?

Having COPD will require you to make some lifestyle changes. If you smoke, you will need to quit. You will also need to avoid places where other people smoke.

To keep your lungs as healthy as possible, you will need to find time to walk or do some other form of exercise daily. If you are not used to exercising, you may find a daily workout very hard at first. The exertion may make you temporarily short of breath. In the long term, however, exercise will make it easier for you to breathe and give you more energy. Talk to your physician about what kind of exercise program is right for you.

With COPD you will not have the stamina you once had. You may need to cut back on activities you used to enjoy. This can lead to frustration, anger, and **depression**. You may benefit from talking with a psychologist or other qualified counselor about your concerns. Ask your physician for referrals or see the organizations listed in the "Resources" section of this book.

Coronary Heart Disease

CORONARY heart disease is the number one killer in the United States. It takes the lives of more than 500,000 Americans each year. Many of those deaths could be prevented. That's because many of the risk factors associated with coronary heart disease—things like smoking, **high blood pressure**, high blood cholesterol, obesity, and physical inactivity—can be controlled. A few risk factors can't be controlled—including age. There's no getting around it: The older you are, the greater your risk for developing heart disease. But no matter what your age, you can reduce your risk by making some healthful lifestyle changes.

Causes

The leading cause of coronary heart disease is *atherosclerosis* (sometimes called "hardening of the arteries"). It occurs when fat and cholesterol, both of which circulate in the blood, build up on the walls of the arteries, narrowing them. The arteries can eventually become so clogged that not enough blood—and oxygen—reaches the heart. The result is coronary heart disease and its complications—*angina, heart attack,*

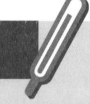

Symptoms

• Tight, squeezing pressure or pain in the center of the chest that lasts for more than a few minutes; it may radiate to the jaw, neck, back, or either arm

• Dizziness or light-headedness

• Shortness of breath

• Sudden onset of rapid heartbeats

• Swelling, particularly in the ankles or lower legs

• Buildup of fluid in the abdomen, lungs, or heart

Important: The symptoms of heart disease differ from person to person. Some people have no symptoms at all. Others have mild chest pain that comes and goes. Still others have strong and steady chest pain.

When to Seek Help

- If you are experiencing crushing or spreading chest pain that may radiate down one or both arms or to the neck or jaw ▶ *Seek emergency care immediately.*

- If you are experiencing sudden shortness of breath, dizziness, nausea, or vomiting, with or without chest pain ▶ *Seek emergency care immediately.*

- If you are experiencing a rapid or uneven heartbeat and feel light-headed or dizzy ▶ *Seek emergency care immediately.*

- If you are experiencing a choking, sharp, or burning pain in the chest, jaw, or abdomen when you rest ▶ *Seek emergency care immediately.*

- If you often experience shortness of breath, even during light activity or while lying down ▶ *Call your nurse information service or physician.*

heart arrhythmia, and *congestive heart failure.* People with high blood cholesterol levels are therefore at higher risk for developing heart disease. So are people who have **high blood pressure** or who smoke. In fact, each of these factors doubles your risk for developing heart disease. And if you have all three risk factors, you are eight times more likely to develop heart disease than someone who has none.

Testing and Treatment

Your doctor may give you one or more diagnostic tests to determine whether you have coronary heart disease. The first test is usually an *electrocardiogram (ECG or EKG)*, which detects electrical abnormalities in the heart. You may also be given a *stress test* (also called a *treadmill test* or *exercise ECG*), which records your heartbeat during exercise. Other tests include *nuclear scanning*, which can reveal damaged areas of your heart, and *coronary angiography*, a test that takes X-rays of blood vessels while the heart is pumping.

Coronary heart disease is often treated with medications and lifestyle changes. Both are important. One of the primary drugs used to relieve the discomfort of coronary heart disease is nitroglycerin. It helps open up the arteries leading to the heart. In severe cases, however, surgery may also be needed. Two common types of heart surgery are *angioplasty*, a procedure that uses a tiny, inflated balloon to reopen closed arteries, and *bypass surgery*, which diverts blood around the same clogged arteries.

> **KNOW THE WARNING SIGNS OF A HEART ATTACK**
>
> **If you or someone else is experiencing any of the following listed symptoms, seek emergency care immediately. Also, take an aspirin to help keep a blood clot from getting bigger. Act quickly. Every minute counts!**
>
> - Uncomfortable pressure, fullness, squeezing, or pain in the center of the chest lasting more than a few minutes.
>
> - Pain that moves from the center of the chest to the shoulders, neck or arms.
>
> - Lightheadedness, fainting, sweating, nausea, or shortness of breath.

Risk Factors

Some of the major risk factors for coronary heart disease can't be changed. But many others can.

Major Risk Factors You *Can't* Change

- Age. The chance of developing heart disease goes up significantly after the age of 65. This is true for both men and women.

- Family history. If heart disease runs in your family, you are more at risk.

- Gender. Men are more likely than women to have a heart attack. And they tend to have them earlier in life. But almost half the people who die of heart attacks each year are women. Heart disease is the leading killer of women as well as of men.

- **Diabetes**. Having **diabetes** seriously increases the risk for developing heart disease. If you have **diabetes**, it is critical that you control other risk factors in addition to controlling your **diabetes**.

Major Risk Factors You *Can* Change

- Smoking. Smoking doubles your risk for having a heart attack. It also greatly increases the odds that you won't survive the heart attack.

- Secondhand smoke. Some evidence indicates that nonsmokers who are frequently exposed to secondhand smoke are at increased risk for heart disease.

- **High blood pressure**. Having high blood pressure can make your heart work harder. Over time, the extra stress on your heart can cause it to enlarge and weaken. This increases your risk for congestive heart failure, heart attack, **stroke**, and kidney failure.

- High blood cholesterol levels. If you are under age 70, the higher your blood cholesterol levels, the higher your risk for heart disease. After age 70, people with low cholesterol have just as many heart attacks as people with high cholesterol.

- Being sedentary. Physical inactivity increases your risk for heart disease.

- Being overweight. People with excess body fat are more likely to develop heart disease and **stroke**. This is true even if they have no other risk factors. The extra pounds appear to put extra strain on the heart.

Women and Heart Disease

Coronary heart disease is not just a man's illness. It strikes women as well—and often with a vengeance. In fact, coronary heart disease is the number one killer of women in the United States. It takes the lives of more than 245,000 women each year—far more than **breast cancer** and lung **cancer** combined.

Each year half a million women have heart attacks. Such attacks are much more deadly for women than for men: Studies have shown that 42 percent of women compared with 24 percent of men die within one year after a heart attack. One reason for the higher death rate may be that the classic symptoms of heart attack tend to look different in women. When a woman has a heart attack, she is more likely to experience nausea, fatigue, and dizziness. As a result, she may not recognize that she is having a heart attack.

The importance of risk factors is also different in women. Non-insulin-dependent **diabetes** tends to be an even stronger contributing risk factor for heart disease in women than in men. So is being overweight.

Surveys have shown that only 30 percent of women talk to their physician about heart disease. Be sure to ask your physician about your risk for this deadly disease. Also, ask how you can keep your heart healthy.

What is...?

...angina? The medical term is *angina pectoris*. It means a choking, suffocating sensation of pain in the chest. But sometimes angina is felt up in the throat and jaws or down one or both arms. Angina happens when the heart doesn't get enough oxygen. The heart may be over-worked, or an artery leading to the heart may be blocked. The pain is similar to that felt during a heart attack, but it doesn't last as long—usually no longer than five minutes. Over time, however, angina can worsen and put you at risk for having a heart attack.

...heart arrhythmia? Also known as an irregular heartbeat, a heart arrhythmia is a disturbance of the normal beating of the heart.

...heart attack? In medical lingo a heart attack is known as a *myocardial infarction*. It literally means "death of heart muscle." A heart attack happens when one of the arteries leading to the heart shuts down, starving the heart of oxygen. The pain is similar to angina but usually lasts for more than 15 minutes and doesn't get better with rest.

...congestive heart failure? This condition happens when the heart no longer pumps at its full capacity. As a result, blood begins to back up in other areas of the body and fluid may accumulate in tissues—especially in the legs and ankles. Sometimes the fluid collects in the lungs. This causes shortness of breath, especially when lying down. Congestive heart failure can lead to death if not treated.

ASPIRIN: SHOULD YOU TAKE IT EVERY DAY?

Taking aspirin regularly can help prevent heart attacks and strokes. It can also reduce the risk for some forms of **cancer**. The protection against heart attacks and **stroke** appears to come from aspirin's ability to keep blood clots from forming.

So should you start taking a daily dose of the familiar white tablet? Not necessarily, say the experts. Like any powerful drug, aspirin has its risks as well as its benefits. Long-term use of aspirin, for example, can lead to bleeding, **stomach ulcers**, gastrointestinal perforations (holes in the stomach or intestines), and a **hearing problem** known as tinnitus.

The American Heart Association recommends that you take an aspirin a day if you have previously had a heart attack or if you have a medical condition that puts you at high risk for a heart attack or **stroke**. Of course, you should always talk to your physician before taking the aspirin.

And what if you don't fit one of those categories and want to take aspirin to prevent a *first* heart attack or **stroke**? That's also a decision you should make only after talking with your physician. He or she will be able to evaluate your individual situation and tell you if the benefits of taking aspirin outweigh the risks for you.

Prevention

- Don't smoke.
- Keep your weight in check. If you are overweight, losing as little as 10 to 20 pounds can help lower your risk for heart disease.
- Exercise regularly. In addition to helping control weight, exercise can help lower blood pressure, relieve stress, and tone the heart and blood vessels.
- Learn how to manage stress.
- Follow a heart-healthy diet. Eat more fruits, vegetables, and whole grains and fewer foods that are salty or high in fat and cholesterol.
- Have a physical examination every one to two years to age 65 and every year after age 65.

- Have your blood pressure checked annually. If you are under age 70, have your cholesterol checked every three to five years.

- Ask your doctor about taking an aspirin a day to prevent heart attack.

KNOW YOUR CHOLESTEROL

Knowing your cholesterol readings can help you and your physician determine your risk for heart disease. But it is only one of many factors. Many people with high cholesterol never get heart disease. In addition, many people who have a heart attack or **stroke** don't have high cholesterol levels. This is especially true of people over age 70. By that age people with low cholesterol have the same risk for having a heart attack as people with high cholesterol. The ability of cholesterol levels to predict heart attacks decreases with age.

To be safe, it's a good idea to have your cholesterol levels checked regularly if you are under the age of 65. (If you're older, ask your physician how often you should have your cholesterol levels checked.) This can be done with a simple blood test at your physician's office. The test's results will include several readings expressed in milligrams per deciliter (mg/dL). Here's how to understand those readings:

• **Total or serum cholesterol.** Total cholesterol below 200 mg/dL is considered desirable; total cholesterol between 200 and 240 is considered borderline; and a level above 240 is high.

• **HDL cholesterol.** HDL, or high-density lipoprotein, is known as the "good cholesterol." High levels of HDL may actually lower the risk for coronary heart disease. Your HDL cholesterol should be 35 mg/dL or higher.

• **LDL cholesterol.** LDL, or low-density lipoprotein, is known as the "bad cholesterol." High levels of LDL have been linked to an increased risk for coronary heart disease. Ideally your LDL level should be below 130 mg/dL. An LDL level between 130 and 160 is considered borderline and a level above 160 is high.

How Will Having Coronary Heart Disease Change My Life?

The diagnosis of heart disease often means stopping or limiting activities until the condition is under control. Once your symptoms are under control, however, you will probably be able to resume most, if not all, of your former activities. Be sure, however, to first get an okay from your physician.

To keep your heart healthy, you may have to change your regular routine. Depending on your current health habits, you may need to quit smoking, exercise more regularly, and change the types of foods you eat. Such changes are difficult because they often require breaking longtime habits. For information and support, contact the American Heart Association and other organizations listed in the "Resources" section of this book.

Diabetes

MEDICAL experts believe that about 16 million people in the United States have diabetes. Yet only half of them know they have it. That's because many people mistake the symptoms of diabetes as signs of aging. As a result, people often don't become aware that they have diabetes until they develop one of its serious and often life-threatening complications. These complications include blindness, kidney disease, nerve disease, **coronary heart disease**, **stroke**, and loss of limbs due to circulatory problems.

Diabetes is a disorder in which the body doesn't produce or properly use *insulin*, a hormone that converts sugar in the muscles to energy. The two main types of diabetes are known as Type 1 and Type 2.

Type 1 diabetes is an autoimmune disease in which the body doesn't produce any insulin. It occurs most often in children and young adults. People with Type 1 diabetes need daily insulin injections to stay alive.

Most—at least 90 percent of—people with diabetes have *Type 2 diabetes*. It is also called *adult-onset diabetes* because it usually develops in

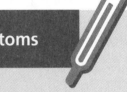

Symptoms

- Extreme thirst
- Continuous need to urinate often, sometimes every hour
- Fatigue and weakness
- Increased appetite
- Weight loss
- Nausea
- Irritability
- Blurred vision
- Repeated or hard-to-heal infections of the skin, gums, vagina, or bladder
- Tingling or loss of feeling in the hands or feet
- Dry, itchy skin

Important: The symptoms of diabetes can be very mild. Older people often mistake them for signs of aging.

adults over the age of 40 and is most common among adults over age 55. Type 2 diabetes is a metabolic disorder in which the body fails to make enough insulin or becomes resistant to the insulin the body does make. Diet and exercise alone can often control this type of diabetes. But some people with Type 2 diabetes also need medicine—either insulin shots or diabetes pills.

Causes

Scientists believe Type 1 diabetes may be triggered by a viral infection. They also suspect that heredity plays a role because Type 1 diabetes tends to run in families.

Genetics may also play a role in Type 2 diabetes because it, too, runs in families. But a primary cause of Type 2 diabetes is being overweight. As people gain weight, their bodies can become more resistant to the effects of insulin.

When to Seek Help

- If your stomach hurts, you feel nauseated and weak, you have excessive thirst, you are urinating very often, you are breathing quickly, and your breath smells sweet

  ▶ *Seek emergency care immediately.*

- If you are very thirsty, weak, tired, sweating, and feel suddenly drowsy or confused

  ▶ *Seek emergency care immediately.*

- If you are experiencing the symptoms of diabetes (opposite)

  ▶ *Call your physician.*

- If you have diabetes and get the **flu**, which can cause your blood sugar levels to go out of control

  ▶ *Call your physician.*

ARE YOU AT RISK?

Find out if you are at risk for having diabetes now. Write in the points next to each statement that is true for you. If a statement is not true, put a zero. Then add your total score.

My weight is equal to or above that listed in the chart opposite.

❏ Yes _____ 5

I am under 65 years of age, and I get little or no exercise during a usual day.

❏ Yes _____ 5

I am between 45 and 64 years old.

❏ Yes _____ 5

I am 65 years old or older.

❏ Yes _____ 9

I am a woman who has had a baby weighing more than 9 pounds.

❏ Yes _____ I

I have a sister or brother with diabetes.

❏ Yes _____ I

I have a parent with diabetes.

❏ Yes _____ I

If you scored 3–9 points:
You are probably at low risk for having diabetes now. But don't just forget about it—especially if you are Hispanic, African American, Native American, Asian American, or Pacific Islander. You may be at higher risk in the future. New guidelines recommend everyone aged 45 and over should consider being tested for the disease every three years.

If you scored 10 or more points:
You are at high risk for having diabetes. Only a doctor can determine whether you have diabetes. See a doctor soon and find out for sure.

Source: American Diabetes Association

Treatment

People with diabetes can live healthy, active lives. The key is to follow a diabetes care plan. That means monitoring your blood sugar levels daily, exercising regularly, maintaining a normal body weight, taking medications as prescribed, managing stress, and seeing your physician for regular checkups. The goal of a diabetes care plan is to keep your blood sugar levels as close to normal as possible. Good control of blood sugar levels can dramatically lower your risk for developing complications.

Your primary care physician will work with you to help you set up a diabetes care plan. He or she may also recommend that you see other health care professionals, including the following:

- an endocrinologist (a physician who specializes in the treatment of diabetes and other disorders of the hormonal system)

- a diabetes nurse educator for instruction in day-to-day care

- a dietitian, for help in planning meals

- an ophthalmologist for eye examinations

- a podiatrist for routine foot care

Living with Diabetes

- Control your weight. Being overweight is the major risk factor for Type 2 diabetes.

- Follow a healthful diet. A low-fat, low-cholesterol diet will help keep your blood sugar and your weight in check. It will also help lower your risk for **coronary heart disease**—a major complication of diabetes.

- Monitor your blood sugar levels. Studies show that people who monitor their blood sugar levels several times daily to achieve "tight control" experience fewer long-term complications.

- Exercise regularly. Exercise can help your body use insulin better. It can also help you keep your weight down. In addition, regular exercise can help lower your blood pressure and cholesterol (and thus your risk for **coronary heart disease**).

- Have regular checkups, including eye exams. It's essential that you and your

AT-RISK WEIGHT CHART

HEIGHT Feet/inches without shoes	WEIGHT Pounds without clothing
4'10"	129
4'11"	133
5'0"	138
5'1"	143
5'2"	147
5'3"	152
5'4"	157
5'5"	162
5'6"	167
5'7"	172
5'8"	177
5'9"	182
5'10"	188
5'11"	193
6'0"	199
6'1"	204
6'2"	210
6'3"	216
6'4"	221

physician work together to monitor your diabetes. Be sure to follow your physician's recommendations for routine checkups and screenings.

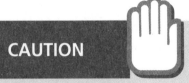

CAUTION

If you have diabetes, you should always wear a medical alert tag. Health care professionals need to be aware of your disease in a medical emergency. Ask your physician about how you can get one.

- Take care of your feet. Foot care is critical for people with diabetes. That's because nerve damage caused by the disease may keep you from feeling pain in your feet. An unnoticed cut or scratch could become infected before you are aware that anything is wrong. Such infections can lead to severe complications, including gangrene. Examine your feet carefully every night. Make sure your shoes fit properly.

- Learn how to better manage the stress in your life. Stress can affect blood sugar. It can also cause you to stop taking care of yourself. Get plenty of rest, stay involved with people, and find moments during your day for relaxation.

How Will Having Diabetes Change My Life?

Your diabetes will require you to make major changes in your daily routine. To manage the disease, you will have to carefully follow a diabetes care plan. For that plan to work you will need to monitor your blood sugar levels, exercise regularly, maintain a normal body weight, take medications as prescribed, manage stress, and see your physician for regular checkups. You may feel alone or set apart from your friends and family because of all this extra work. You may also feel under constant danger—of insulin reactions or complications. Men with diabetes often have the added problem of impotence, a common side effect of the disease.

It's not uncommon for people with diabetes to have feelings of frustration, anger, and **depression** from time to time. If you are experiencing such feelings, you may benefit from talking with a psychologist or other qualified counselor. You may also want to consider joining a support group for people with diabetes. Ask your physician for referrals, or contact the American Diabetes Association or other organizations listed in the "Resources" section of this book.

Diverticular Disorders: Diverticulosis and Diverticulitis

MANY people over age 50 have small pouches that bulge outward from weak spots in their colon (the major part of the large intestine). These pouches are called *diverticula*. The condition of having them is called *diverticulosis*.

Diverticulosis is fairly harmless. But sometimes the pouches become inflamed—a more serious condition called *diverticulitis*. It can lead to infections, internal bleeding, or blockages in the colon and other complications. Diverticulitis must be treated to make sure it doesn't become a life-threatening illness.

Causes

A low-fiber diet seems to be the major cause of diverticular disorders. Fiber makes stools soft and easy to pass. Not eating enough fiber can cause **constipation**. People who are constipated must strain to move a stool that is too hard. This puts increased pressure on the colon—pressure that can cause diverticular pouches to form. If the pouches then become filled with undigested food, they may become infected and inflamed.

Symptoms

DIVERTICULOSIS

- Mild cramps

- Bloating

- **Constipation**

Important: Most people with diverticulosis have no symptoms.

DIVERTICULITIS

- Abdominal pain, especially on the lower left side of the abdomen

- Nausea or vomiting

- Fever

- **Constipation**

Treatment

Your physician may have you eat more high-fiber foods to prevent **constipation**. For a mild case of diverticulitis, your physician may prescribe bed rest, stool softeners, a liquid diet, and antibiotics or other drugs. Serious cases of diverticulitis sometimes require hospitalization, intravenous antibiotics, and even surgery.

Prevention

- Eat more fiber. (For good food sources of fiber, see p. 5.)

- Drink more fluids—at least eight glasses of water each day.

- Exercise regularly.

- Don't ignore the urge to have a bowel movement.

- Avoid straining during a bowel movement.

- Don't use laxatives unless your physician advises them. Overuse of laxatives can cause **constipation**.

When to Seek Help

- If you have sharp abdominal pain or swelling, fever, chills, and nausea or vomiting

Seek emergency care immediately.

How Will Having Diverticulitis Change My Life?

Once your symptoms are under control, you should be able to resume most, if not all, of your former activities. To keep the infection from happening again, however, you may need to make some lifestyle changes. These may include eating more fiber, drinking more water, and exercising more regularly.

High Blood Pressure (Hypertension)

As blood flows from the heart, it creates pressure against the walls of the blood vessels. The harder the heart is working, the greater the pressure. Too much pressure—or high blood pressure—can eventually damage the vessels. That can lead to serious health problems, including vision loss, **stroke**, **coronary heart disease**, and kidney failure. In the elderly, high blood pressure can cause congestive heart failure.

High blood pressure, or *hypertension*, is very common among adults in the United States: One in four adults has it. Yet almost one-third of people with high blood pressure don't know they have it. (That figure is believed to be even higher among older adults.) The reason: High blood pressure rarely shows any symptoms. People who have high blood pressure often feel fine—until they experience one of the disease's serious consequences. That's why high blood pressure is often called "the silent killer."

Symptoms

Most people with high blood pressure have no symptoms. People with severe high blood pressure may have the following symptoms:

- Dizziness
- Persistent **headaches**
- Nosebleeds
- Confusion

Causes

In as many as 95 percent of cases of high blood pressure, the cause is unknown. This type of high blood pressure is called *essential hypertension*. Certain risk factors have been linked to essential hypertension, including being overweight, drinking too much alcohol, and possibly eating too much salt. Heredity also plays a role, as do age and race. Your risk for having high blood pressure increases as you age. And African Americans are more likely to have high blood pressure than white Americans.

A very small percentage of cases of high blood pressure is caused by other illnesses, such as kidney disease. This type of high blood pressure is called *secondary hypertension.*

Treatment

Secondary hypertension can often be cured by treating the underlying cause. Essential hypertension can't be cured, but it can be kept under control. If you have

When to Seek Help

- If you have high blood pressure and experience a sudden onset of confusion
  ▶ *Seek emergency care immediately.*

- If you have high blood pressure and experience any symptoms of severe high blood pressure (p. 91)
  ▶ *Seek emergency care.*

- If you are taking an antihypertensive drug and experience side effects, such as drowsiness, constipation, dizziness, or loss of sexual function
  ▶ *Seek emergency care.*

- If you have checked your blood pressure several times in a given week and the average reading is greater than 140/90 despite lifestyle changes and/or medication
  ▶ *Call your nurse information service or physician.*

mild high blood pressure, your physician may recommend that you lose weight, exercise more, cut down on alcohol and salt, and practice relaxation techniques such as yoga or meditation to reduce stress.

Some cases of high blood pressure require medication. Among the drugs commonly prescribed are diuretics and beta-blockers. Diuretics flush excess fluid out of the body. This reduces the amount of fluid in the blood and allows small arteries to relax. Beta-blockers help the heart beat more slowly and with less force. Other medications for high blood pressure include angiotensin antagonists, angiotensin converting enzyme (ACE) inhibitors, calcium channel-blockers (CCBs), alpha-blockers, alpha/beta-blockers, nervous system inhibitors, and vasodilators. These drugs help blood vessels relax and pressure to go down. Your physician will choose the drug—or drugs—that will work best for you.

Prevention

- If you smoke, stop.

- Maintain a healthy weight. If you are overweight, losing even a few pounds may make a big difference in preventing high blood pressure.

- Become more physically active.

- Watch what you eat. Make sure your daily diet includes lots of fresh fruit, vegetables, and whole grains. Cut back on foods that are high in fat, cholesterol, and calories.

- If you drink alcohol, do so in moderation.

- Learn better ways of coping with stress.

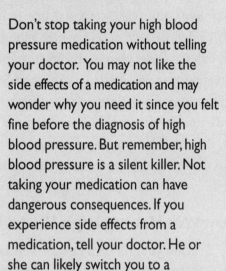

CAUTION

Don't stop taking your high blood pressure medication without telling your doctor. You may not like the side effects of a medication and may wonder why you need it since you felt fine before the diagnosis of high blood pressure. But remember, high blood pressure is a silent killer. Not taking your medication can have dangerous consequences. If you experience side effects from a medication, tell your doctor. He or she can likely switch you to a different drug that can control your blood pressure without affecting your quality of life.

Get Your Blood Pressure Checked Regularly

You should have your blood pressure checked at least once a year. It's a quick, safe, and painless test. Blood pressure readings are given in two numbers. The first number indicates *systolic pressure*. This is the force with which the heart pumps blood into the arteries. The second number is the *diastolic pressure*. This is the pressure between heartbeats, or when the heart is relaxed. That's why it's always a lower number.

Blood pressure is measured in millimeters of mercury, which is abbreviated mm Hg. A normal healthy blood pressure reading is about 120/80 mm Hg. But the definition of normal depends on age, gender, general health, and other factors. A slightly higher or slightly lower reading for either number may not be a problem. A reading of 140/90 is considered a sign of high blood pressure. Some type of treatment—lifestyle changes, drugs, or both—may be needed. A reading of 180/110 is considered a sign of severe high blood pressure. It requires immediate treatment.

Often in older people, the first number (systolic pressure) is high while the second (diastolic pressure) is normal. This condition is called *isolated systolic hypertension.* It requires treatment. Research has shown that older people can reduce their risk for **stroke** and heart attack by lowering their systolic blood pressure.

Because blood pressure can vary over the course of a day, you should have it tested more than once if you get a high reading. Many things can affect blood pressure—including worrying about having it tested!

How Will Having High Blood Pressure Change My Life?

To lower your blood pressure—and keep it there—you may have to make major lifestyle changes. You may need to quit smoking, limit your alcohol consumption, exercise more regularly, learn to manage stress, and change the types of foods you eat. Such changes are difficult because they often require breaking longtime habits. For information and support, contact the American Heart Association and other organizations listed in the "Resources" section of this book.

HIV and AIDS

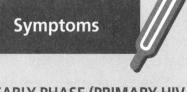

AIDS (acquired immune deficiency syndrome) is a serious, usually fatal disease of the immune system. It is believed to be caused by HIV (human immunodeficiency virus). HIV attacks the body's immune system, leaving it unable to fight off bacteria, viruses, and other microbes. People with AIDS usually die from **cancer**, **pneumonia**, or some other infection.

Symptoms

EARLY PHASE (PRIMARY HIV INFECTION)

- Flulike symptoms, such as fever, fatigue, muscle and joint pain, **headaches**, and sore throat. These symptoms can last from three days to more than a month. Most people then enter a symptom-free phase that can last 5 to 10 years or longer.

Important: Many people with primary HIV infection have few or no symptoms.

AS HIV PROGRESSES TO AIDS

- Swollen glands in the neck, armpits, or groin
- Long-term fatigue
- Fever, chills, and night sweats
- Unexplained weight loss
- Cough and shortness of breath
- Severe **headaches**
- Chronic diarrhea
- White patches in the mouth (thrush)
- Bruises or skin sores that do not clear up
- Yeast infections that do not go away after treatment
- Changes in vision
- Finally, severe infections, cancers, and various illnesses of the lungs, heart, digestive system, and central nervous system. Also, confusion, loss of memory, and personality changes.

HIV is found in blood, semen, and vaginal secretions and sometimes in breast milk. It is spread mostly through unprotected sexual contact and by sharing injection needles. In addition, mothers infected with HIV can transmit the virus to their babies, either during pregnancy or birth or through breast milk. The virus can also be spread through contaminated blood transfusions, but all donated blood in the United States is now tested for HIV before it is used.

HIV *cannot* be transmitted by casual contact. For example, you don't get HIV from kissing or hugging an infected person. Nor do you get it by sharing a glass of water, a swimming pool, or bedding with an infected person.

Although young adults are at the greatest risk for contracting HIV and AIDS, more than 10 percent of people with AIDS in the United States are over the age of 50. And researchers report that the number of older adults infected with HIV is increasing.

Treatment

There is no cure for AIDS. Nor is there a vaccine. But new treatments—some combining several drugs—have been developed that can fight both the HIV infection and its associated infections and cancers. These treatments have made it

When to Seek Help

- If you have been exposed to HIV infection through sex with an infected person or by sharing hypodermic needles

▶ *Seek emergency care immediately.*

- If you experience symptoms of HIV infection (see p. 95)

▶ *Call your nurse information service or physician.*

- If you have HIV or AIDS and your symptoms get worse or you have a new symptom

▶ *Call your physician.*

possible for infected people to live longer, healthier lives. Talk to your physician about the latest advances in AIDS treatments. You can also keep up-to-date on AIDS treatments and research through the organizations listed in the "Resources" section of this book.

Getting Tested

The only way to tell if you have been infected with HIV is to be tested. The test involves taking a blood sample to see if your body is producing antibodies to the virus. If you think you may have been exposed to the virus, call your physician immediately. Many communities also have anonymous HIV counseling and testing centers. You can find these centers by calling your local or state health department.

If you test positive, it's extremely important that your sexual partners be told of the diagnosis. They will also need to be tested.

Prevention

- Practice safer sex. Use a latex condom (even during oral sex) unless you are certain that both you and your partner are not infected.

- Don't use illegal drugs. Sharing contaminated needles spreads AIDS.

- Don't come in blood-to-blood contact with another person.

- If you continue engaging in activities that put you at high risk for HIV infection, you and your partner(s) should be tested every 6 to 12 months.

How Will Having an HIV Infection Change My Life?

Living with an HIV infection will have a profound effect on your life. When you first learn of the diagnosis, you may feel shock, panic, and anger. You may find it difficult to believe what has happened to you. These are very normal reactions. It can take time to accept HIV.

Many people in the early stages of an HIV infection appear in good health. But even if you feel fine, it's important that you get regular medical checkups and tests to measure your health. You will need to make significant lifestyle changes to take care of both your physical and emotional health and to keep from developing a secondary infection. These changes include eating nutritiously and taking all medications precisely as prescribed by your physician. You'll need to take your dosages on a very strict timetable. This will help you avoid developing a resistance to different kinds of HIV medications and will maximize the effectiveness of the drugs. You may also need to change your sexual activities so as not to put others at risk for contracting the disease.

Living with HIV can be lonely. But you don't have to deal with it alone. Fortunately many organizations offer support to people with HIV or AIDS. Ask your physician for referrals, or contact the organizations listed in the "Resources" section of this book.

Osteoporosis

OSTEOPOROSIS, which means "porous bones," is a condition in which bones gradually weaken and thin. This leaves the bones more vulnerable to breaks or fractures—especially in the hip, spine, and wrist. Each year osteoporosis leads to 1.5 million fractures, including 300,000 hip fractures. For elderly people, breaking a hip can be particularly dangerous. That's because treatment for a hip fracture requires being immobile in bed for a long period of time. Immobility increases the risk for developing **pneumonia** or a blood clot.

Most people don't know they have osteoporosis until they have a fracture. Yet osteoporosis is very common. More than 28 million Americans are believed to have the condition.

Causes

Calcium is the mineral that makes bones hard. Starting around the time you reach age 35, your bones begin to lose calcium faster than they can replace it. Scientists don't fully understand exactly what causes the excessive thinning and weakening of the bones, known as osteoporosis. But they have identified many factors that can put you at risk for the condition:

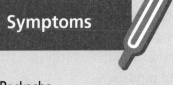

Symptoms

- Backache
- Fracture of the wrist, hip, or spine
- Gradual loss of height and stooped posture
- Loss of bone in the jaw

Important: Most people with osteoporosis have no symptoms until they fracture a bone.

- Age. Bones tend to become less dense and weaker as you age.

- Gender. Most people with osteoporosis (80 percent) are women. The condition is uncommon in men until after age 70. Women are more at risk because they generally have less bone tissue than men and because they tend to lose bone quickly in the years right after menopause. Researchers believe this rapid bone loss may be linked to falling estrogen levels.

- Race. White and Asian women are more likely to develop osteoporosis than Hispanic and African American women.

- Family history. Women with a family history of osteoporosis are more at risk.

- Body frame and weight. If you are small boned and thin, you are at greater risk.

- Menopause history. The earlier you experienced **menopause**, the greater your risk. This is especially true of women who have had "surgical **menopause**"— removal of their ovaries—before age 40.

- Medications. Taking certain medications, such as corticosteroids, can increase your risk.

- Illnesses. Several medical conditions, including rheumatoid **arthritis** and an overactive thyroid, can increase your risk.

Diagnosis

Several tests are used to detect osteoporosis. The most widely used is *dual energy X-ray absorptiometry (DEXA)*. It measures bone density in the wrist, hip, and lower spine. If you think you are at risk for osteoporosis, discuss this and other tests with your physician.

When to Seek Help

- If you have a fall or accident that may have caused a bone fracture ▶ *Seek emergency care immediately.*

- If you develop sudden, severe back pain or a persistent backache ▶ *Call your nurse information service or physician.*

- If you have risk factors for osteoporosis ▶ *Call your nurse information service or physician.*

ARE YOU AT RISK?

Listed below are questions that identify women at risk for developing osteoporosis. If you answer "Yes" to many of these questions, talk to your physician about ways you can reduce your risk.

Do you have a small or thin frame?
☐ Yes ☐ No

Are you Caucasian or Asian?
☐ Yes ☐ No

Has a member of your family been diagnosed with osteoporosis?
☐ Yes ☐ No

Did you reach **menopause** before age 40, or was **menopause** surgically induced?
☐ Yes ☐ No

Have you taken thyroid medication for an extended period of time?
☐ Yes ☐ No

Have you taken high doses of cortisonelike drugs for asthma, **arthritis**, or **cancer**?
☐ Yes ☐ No

During childhood, was your diet low in dairy products and other sources of calcium?
☐ Yes ☐ No

Today, is your diet low in dairy products and other sources of calcium?
☐ Yes ☐ No

Is your diet high in salt, caffeine, or protein?
☐ Yes ☐ No

Are you physically inactive?
☐ Yes ☐ No

Do you smoke?
☐ Yes ☐ No

Do you drink alcohol heavily now, or did you drink heavily in the past?
☐ Yes ☐ No

Did you have *amenorrhea* (lack of menstrual periods for an extended amount of time)?
☐ Yes ☐ No

Have you ever been diagnosed with anorexia?
☐ Yes ☐ No

Source: University of Pennsylvania Health System

Treatment

Treatment for osteoporosis has two purposes: to stop further bone loss and to prevent falls that can cause fractures. To slow down bone loss, your physician may suggest that you increase the amount of calcium in your diet or perhaps take calcium supplements. Your physician may also recommend a vitamin D supplement. Your body needs vitamin D to absorb calcium. You can absorb enough vitamin D by being outside for as little as 10 minutes every day. But if you aren't outside enough, you may need a supplement. In addition, your physician may encourage you to begin a regular exercise program—one specially designed for people with osteoporosis.

Did You Know?

Here's an easy way to get more calcium into your diet: Add nonfat dry milk to soups, casseroles, beverages, and other foods. Each teaspoon of dry milk has about 20 mg of calcium.

Several medications are available for the prevention and treatment of osteoporosis.

- Estrogen replacement therapy (ERT) (for women only). Studies have shown that women who begin ERT soon after **menopause** have fewer hip and wrist fractures later in life. The estrogen must be taken indefinitely, however, because once the medication is stopped, bone begins to thin again. ERT is not without its health risks, including an increased risk for uterine and breast cancers. (For more information, see pp. 210-211.)

- Calcitonin. This naturally occurring hormone has been shown to slow bone loss. It may also relieve the pain associated with bone fractures. Calcitonin cannot be taken orally; it is available as an injection or nasal spray.

- Bisphosphonates. These compounds have also been shown to increase bone density and reduce the risk for hip and spine fractures.

- Selective estrogen receptor modulators (SERMs). These are compounds that have estrogenlike effects on the body. They appear to prevent bone loss throughout the body. Unlike estrogens, SERMs don't appear to stimulate uterine or breast tissue.

Preventing a fall, which could cause a bone fracture, is also an important part of treating osteoporosis. Take steps to ensure your environment is safe from falls (see p. 321.) Regular exercise can also help prevent falls by increasing your muscle strength, coordination, and flexibility. In addition, be sure to have your eyesight checked regularly. Poor eyesight, if uncorrected, can cause you to trip and fall.

Prevention

- Don't smoke. Smoking appears to increase the risk for osteoporosis.

- Reduce your use of alcohol. Too much alcohol appears to increase the risk for osteoporosis. Using alcohol also increases your risk for injuries that may cause fractures.

- Reduce your use of caffeine. Caffeine may increase the amount of calcium that is excreted in urine. This may weaken bones.

- Exercise regularly. Be sure the exercise is weight bearing and that it strengthens both the upper and lower body.

- Eat foods rich in calcium. Also, consider taking a calcium supplement.

How Will Having Osteoporosis Change My Life?

Having osteoporosis may not necessarily change your daily routine. But fracturing a bone—a common side effect of osteoporosis—will. Breaking a bone can greatly limit your movement—and your daily activities. If you fracture a hip, you will be hospitalized. Recovery from a hip fracture is often long and difficult.

Osteoporosis may eventually cause the bones in your back to break. You may then experience loss of height, back pain, and a curvature of the spine, commonly known as a "dowager's hump."

If you have osteoporosis, you'll need to make some lifestyle changes to prevent further bone loss. These changes include taking time every day to exercise. Be sure your exercise program is approved by your physician. You'll probably be told to avoid any activity that puts sudden or excessive strain on your bones. Also, be careful when lifting heavy things, like a bag of groceries.

To prevent fractures, you'll need to take steps to prevent falls. This may mean rearranging your living space—getting rid of throw rugs, for example, and installing hand railings. For more information about living with osteoporosis, contact the National Osteoporosis Foundation (p. 343).

Parkinson's Disease

PARKINSON'S disease is a chronic, progressive disorder of the central nervous system. It affects about 1.5 million Americans. The disease can start at any age, but it usually begins between the ages of 50 and 65. It is slightly more common in men than in women.

Symptoms differ from person to person. One early symptom of the disease is weakness or stiffness in an arm or leg. Another early symptom is a slight tremor of a hand when it's at rest. (Movement usually stops the tremor.) Eventually the stiffness and shaking worsen. It becomes harder to maintain balance and coordination. Everyday activities, such as walking, getting out of a chair, and speaking, can become a struggle. This can lead to **depression** or other emotional responses.

Symptoms

PRIMARY SYMPTOMS

- Rigidity, or stiffness, of arms, legs, or neck
- Tremors, mostly in the hands when they are at rest
- Poor balance
- Slowness in movement
- Shuffling walk

SECONDARY SYMPTOMS

- **Depression**
- Sleep disturbances
- Dizziness
- Stooped posture
- **Constipation**
- Dementia
- Problems with speech, breathing, swallowing, and sexual function

Causes

The symptoms of Parkinson's disease are caused by the loss of cells in an area of the brain known as the *substantia nigra*. These cells are needed to produce a chemical called *dopamine*, which helps people move normally and smoothly. People with Parkinson's don't make enough dopamine in their brains.

Scientists don't know exactly what causes the cells in the substantia nigra to become damaged. A defective gene may be at fault in a few cases. But researchers believe that genetic factors alone are not responsible for most cases of Parkinson's. They suspect that Parkinson's results from a combination of factors. One factor may be a genetic predisposition to the disease. Another might be exposure to an environmental trigger—perhaps a virus or a chemical toxin.

When to Seek Help

- If you are experiencing the symptoms of Parkinson's disease (opposite)

▼

Call your nurse information service or physician.

Treatment

There is no cure for Parkinson's disease. But the symptoms can be controlled—sometimes for years—with medications or surgery. Commonly prescribed medications include levodopa, anticholinergics, Selegiline, dopamine agonists, and COMT inhibitors. All of these drugs add either dopamine or dopaminelike chemicals to the brain.

Surgery can also help some people control their symptoms. A type of surgery known as a *pallidotomy* uses an electrode to destroy the brain cells that are causing unwanted tremors. Another type of surgery—*deep brain stimulation*—implants a device in the brain. The patient can switch the device on or off when needed to control tremors.

Living with Parkinson's Disease

- Exercise regularly. Research has also shown that Parkinson's tends to progress more slowly in people who stay active. Staying active will also help you ward off **depression** and many of the other secondary symptoms of Parkinson's. Continue those activities you enjoyed before your disease was diagnosed. Or find new ones that interest you and bring you pleasure.

- Join a support group. Sharing your feelings and frustrations about your Parkinson's disease can make living with this chronic disease easier. A support group can help you realize that you aren't alone, and it can provide you with many helpful ideas and resources. Your physician or your local chapter of the Parkinson's Disease Association can help you find a support group near you.

How Will Having Parkinson's Disease Change My Life?

Living with Parkinson's disease is a different experience for each person who has it. That's because the disease's progress and symptoms vary from person to person. But you should expect to experience many changes.

Parkinson's disease often begins with a tremor of the hand on one side of the body. You may notice some slowness and stiffness on the affected side. Eventually, doing everyday tasks that require finger and hand coordination, such as brushing teeth, shaving, and buttoning clothes, may become more difficult.

Walking may also begin to take great effort. Your steps may become shorter, and the foot on the affected side of the body may drag. You may also experience episodes of feeling "stuck in place" when trying to walk, a symptom known as "freezing."

As the disease progresses, you may lose some facial expression and your eyes may blink less often. In addition, your voice may become lower and flat in tone.

Having Parkinson's disease is a physical and emotional challenge. It can affect your self-image and lead to frustration, anger, and **depression**. Adjusting to living with the disease takes time and patience. You may benefit from talking with a psychologist or other qualified counselor about your concerns. Ask your physician for referrals.

You may also want to consider joining a support group for people who are going through a similar experience with Parkinson's disease. Ask your physician for referrals, or contact the organizations listed in the "Resources" section of this book.

Stroke

A stroke is sometimes called a "brain attack." It happens when there is a sudden stoppage of blood flow to the brain. Blood carries much needed oxygen and other nutrients to the brain's cells. When the flow of blood shuts down, the cells become damaged and die, usually within minutes. As the cells die, you may lose your ability to speak, walk, think, and breathe.

About 500,000 Americans have strokes each year. More than 145,000 people die annually from stroke-related causes. That makes stroke the third leading killer in the United States, right behind **coronary heart disease** and **cancer**.

Although some people recover fully after a stroke, most have some kind of lasting physical or mental disability. In fact, stroke is the most common cause of disability in adults. It is second only to **Alzheimer's disease** as a cause of dementia.

Causes

Strokes can occur when a blood clot blocks an artery in the brain or in the neck. These are called *ischemic strokes.* Most strokes (about 80 percent) fall into this category. Less

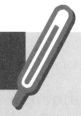

Symptoms

- Sudden numbness or weakness of face, arm, or leg—especially on one side of the body

- Sudden confusion, trouble speaking or understanding

- Sudden trouble seeing in one or both eyes

- Sudden trouble walking, dizziness, loss of balance, or coordination

- Sudden severe **headaches** with no known cause

Important: Sometimes stroke symptoms last only a few minutes and disappear. This may be a sign of a *transient ischemic attack (TIA).* Don't ignore one of these "ministrokes." It can be a forerunner to a future, full-blown stroke.

When to Seek Help

- If you are experiencing any of the symptoms of stroke (p. 107)   ▶ *Seek emergency care immediately.*

- If you have experienced any of these symptoms in the past   ▶ *See your physician.*

common are *hemorrhagic strokes.* These are caused when an artery in the brain bursts and begins bleeding.

Treatment

Strokes are medical emergencies. If you think you or someone you know is having a stroke, seek emergency medical care immediately. Every minute counts. You may be given drugs to dissolve blood clots and lower blood pressure.

After the stroke, you'll need treatment to prevent future strokes. Your physician will talk to you about making diet, exercise, and other lifestyle changes to lower your risk. You'll also need ongoing drug treatment. You may be given blood thinners or anticoagulants to help keep new blood clots from forming or antihypertensive medications to lower your blood pressure. Aspirin is sometimes prescribed to protect against ischemic strokes. Your physician may also recommend surgery to open clogged arteries.

Recovering from a Stroke

A crucial part of treatment for stroke is rehabilitation. Although stroke permanently destroys brain cells, it is possible to "train" other cells to take over certain functions, such as speech or muscle movement. Stroke rehabilitation should begin as soon as possible—often before leaving the hospital. Rehabilitation usually includes the following therapies:

- Physical therapy to strengthen muscles and improve balance and coordination

- Speech and language therapy to relearn how to talk and communicate

- Occupational therapy to improve eye-hand coordination and skills needed for everyday tasks, such as bathing and cooking

- Support and counseling to help adjust to the physical and emotional changes that follow a stroke

Your physician will refer you to stroke rehabilitation specialists. You can also get helpful information from the organizations listed in the "Resources" section of this book.

Risk Factors

Some of the major risk factors for stroke can't be changed. But many others can.

Major Risk Factors You *Can't* Change

- Age. The chance of developing a stroke goes up significantly after the age of 60. This is true for both men and women.

- Family history. If a parent or sibling had a stroke, you are more at risk.

- Gender. Men are more likely than women to have a stroke.

- Race. African Americans are 2 to 3 times more likely to have an ischemic stroke and $2^1/_2$ times more likely to die from it than white Americans.

- **Diabetes.** Having **diabetes** seriously increases the risk for having a stroke. If you have **diabetes**, it is critical that you control other risk factors as well as your **diabetes**.

Major Risk Factors You *Can* Change

- **High blood pressure.** This is the leading cause of strokes.

- Smoking. Smoking doubles your risk for having a stroke.

- High blood cholesterol levels. The higher your blood cholesterol levels, the greater your risk for stroke.

- **Coronary heart disease.** Having heart disease can increase the chances of a blood clot forming.

- Being sedentary. Physical inactivity increases your risk for stroke.

- Being overweight. People with excess body fat are more likely to have a stroke.

Prevention

- Don't smoke. Your risk for stroke drops dramatically within a few years of stopping smoking.

> ### A NOTE TO CAREGIVERS
>
> Taking care of a loved one who has had a stroke can be stressful. Fortunately there are many good resources available for family caregivers of stroke survivors. The organizations listed in the "Resources" section of this book are a good place to start. Also, see "10 Tips for Family Caregivers" on pp. 56-57.

- Control your blood pressure. Have your blood pressure checked annually. If it is high, follow your physician's advice on how to lower it.

- Have your cholesterol checked every three to five years.

- Keep your weight in check.

- Exercise regularly. In addition to helping control weight, exercise can help lower blood pressure, relieve stress, and tone the heart and blood vessels.

- Learn how to manage stress.

- Follow a healthful diet. Eat more fruits, vegetables, and whole grains and fewer foods that are salty or high in fat and cholesterol.

- Ask your doctor about taking an aspirin a day to prevent stroke.

How Will Having a Stroke Change My Life?

Recovery from a stroke takes time and effort. Your physician will have you begin rehabilitation as soon as your condition is stable. You may need to learn many basic skills all over again. How quickly and completely you recover from a stroke depends on many factors, including your age and the severity of your stroke. Some people recover from a stroke within weeks; others take months or even years. Some people never fully recover all their former abilities.

You may notice that your emotional responses are different after your stroke, particularly within the first few weeks. It is common for stroke survivors to have rapid mood changes. You may start crying one moment and then start laughing the next. You may also become depressed. In fact, one-third to one-half of all survivors experience **depression** within months of their stroke. These responses are often the direct result of the injury to the brain.

Adjusting to life after a stroke can also lead to intense emotions. As you struggle to recover, you may experience feelings of frustration, **anxiety**, anger, apathy, and sadness. These feelings are understandable. But if they persist, you should seek help from a psychologist or other qualified counselor. Ask your physician for referrals. You may also want to consider joining a support group for stroke survivors. Ask your physician for referrals, or contact the organizations listed in the "Resources" section of this book.

Thyroid Problems

THE thyroid is a small, butterfly-shaped gland located in the neck, right below the larynx (Adam's apple). It makes hormones that play a role in all functions of the body, including how fast your body absorbs food and turns it into energy.

Symptoms

HYPERTHYROIDISM (INCREASED THYROID ACTIVITY)

- Weight loss despite increased appetite
- Nervousness, irritability
- Rapid heartbeat
- Increased sweating
- Difficulty sleeping
- More frequent bowel movements
- Muscle weakness, shaky hands
- Goiter (swelling of the thyroid gland in the front of the neck)
- **Hair loss**
- Bulging, watery eyes

HYPOTHYROIDISM (DECREASED THYROID ACTIVITY)

- Fatigue, muscle aches
- Feeling cold too easily
- Dry skin and hair, brittle nails
- **Constipation**
- Forgetfulness
- Weight gain for no reason
- Puffy face
- Goiter (swelling of the thyroid gland in the front of the neck)
- **Depression**

About 20 million Americans have some kind of thyroid disease. Thyroid problems are common among older people—particularly among older women. Yet many people with these conditions don't know they have them. The symptoms, which can include fatigue, dry skin, hair loss, and forgetfulness, are often overlooked. People mistakenly think these are "just part of getting old."

The most common thyroid problems are the following:

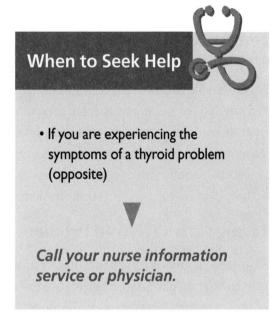

When to Seek Help

• If you are experiencing the symptoms of a thyroid problem (opposite)

▼

Call your nurse information service or physician.

- *Hyperthyroidism.* People with this condition have an overactive thyroid: It makes too much thyroid hormone. As a result, the body speeds up. By age 60 about 17 percent of women and 9 percent of men have higher than normal levels of thyroid hormone.

- *Hypothyroidism.* People with this condition have an underactive thyroid: Their thyroid gland either makes too little thyroid hormone, or the body can't respond to the hormone it does make. As a result, the body slows down. Up to 16 percent of people over the age of 60 have an underactive thyroid.

Causes

Graves' disease, an autoimmune disorder, is the most common cause of hyperthyroidism. In Graves' disease, the thyroid is attacked in a way that makes it produce too much thyroid hormone. Other causes of hyperthyroidism include benign tumors and viral infections.

Hypothyroidism is also caused by an autoimmune disorder that attacks and destroys the thyroid gland. Radiation and certain drugs (including those for hyperthyroidism) can cause hypothyroidism as well.

Diagnosis and Treatment

A simple blood test can determine if your thyroid is making too little or too much thyroid hormone. Treatment for hyperthyroidism usually includes radioactive iodine, an antithyroid medication, or surgery. If you have hypothyroidism, your physician will probably prescribe a thyroid hormone supplement. Each of these treatments is aimed at disabling the thyroid gland.

Some people with overactive or underactive thyroids develop **vision problems**. To help protect your vision, your physician may refer you to an ophthalmologist.

Living with a Thyroid Problem

- Exercise regularly. Do 20 minutes or more of aerobic exercise each day. It can help your thyroid gland work better. Be sure to talk with your physician, however, before starting an exercise program.

- If you smoke, stop. Smoking can make **vision problems** worse.

- Take care of your eyes. Get regular eye exams. If your eyes feel dry, moisten them with over-the-counter or prescription artificial tears. If they are red and swollen in the morning, try sleeping with your head raised. If your eyelids cannot close completely, wear eye patches while sleeping. The patches will help keep your corneas from drying out. Also, wear sunglasses during the day to protect your eyes from bright light and wind.

How Will Having a Thyroid Problem Change My Life?

Once your symptoms are under control, you should be able to resume your former activities. You will need to have your thyroid levels checked regularly by your physician, however, for the rest of your life. You will also need to get regular eye exams with an ophthalmologist.

Common Health Problems

Most health problems are not life-threatening. You develop a **cold** or a **headache**. You pull a back muscle or have trouble sleeping. Usually such problems can be easily treated, sometimes by following a few simple self-care measures.

Yet many common, everyday health problems can develop into more serious concerns. This is particularly true for older people. The **flu** may develop into **pneumonia**, for example. Or a **urinary tract infection** may lead to permanent kidney damage. That's why it's so important to pay attention to your body and your health. Know when to stop and take care of yourself—and when to seek medical care. Practice preventive care. By taking such actions you can lower the risk of having a minor ailment develop into a major or chronic health problem.

Sometimes, what may seem like a minor health problem is actually a symptom of a more serious, underlying illness. Or it may indicate a reaction to medication. If you have a health problem that persists or keeps recurring—a bad **cold**, for example, or a **headache**—be sure to tell your doctor about it. Chances are good that nothing more sinister is afoot. But it's always best to check with your doctor.

Of course, just because a health problem isn't life-threatening, doesn't mean it won't have a major impact on your quality of life. **Incontinence** is not in itself a serious illness, for example, but it can severely curtail your everyday activities. And **hearing problems** and **vision problems**—common concerns for older people—can have a tremendous impact on how you interact with the world around you. But again, in most cases these problems can be successfully treated and you can return to living an active, productive life.

On the following pages, you'll find some of the more common health problems that affect people aged 50 and older.

Back and Neck Problems

MOST people develop back or neck problems at some time during their life. In fact, back pain, especially lower back pain, is one of the most common reasons people go to see a physician.

Back and neck problems can take many forms, such as sprained ligaments, strained muscles, ruptured disks, irritated joints, or compression fractures (the result of the bone-thinning condition known as **osteoporosis**). The pain or discomfort can be acute (coming on suddenly and lasting only a few days to several weeks). Or it can be chronic (lasting longer than three months).

Causes

Back and neck problems are usually caused by bad habits, such as poor posture, lack of exercise, or lifting things carelessly. Obesity can also lead to back or neck problems. So can stress. In older people, decades of "wear and tear" as well as **arthritis** and **osteoporosis** can lead to back and neck pain. Several illnesses and conditions can also trigger such pain, including **bladder infections**, kidney stones, kidney infections, and blood clots.

Symptoms

- Constant pain or stiffness anywhere along the spine, from the neck to the hips

- Sharp pain in the neck, upper back, or lower back, especially after lifting a heavy object or doing something else that is physically strenuous

- Chronic ache in the middle or lower back, especially after sitting or standing for a long period of time

- Chronic back pain when walking

When to Seek Help

- If you have a stiff neck that is accompanied by headache and fever

  ▶ *Seek emergency care immediately.*

- If you have severe neck pain or severe back pain across the upper back that came on suddenly for no apparent reason

  ▶ *Seek emergency care immediately.*

- If you have back pain that is accompanied by the sudden onset of bladder or bowel control trouble

  ▶ *Seek emergency care immediately.*

- If you have neck or back pain that comes on gradually and is accompanied by pain that radiates down the arms or legs

  ▶ *Call your nurse information service or physician.*

- If you have neck or back pain that is accompanied by numbness, tingling, or weakness in the feet or toes

  ▶ *Call your nurse information service or physician.*

- If you have neck or back pain that is keeping you from doing your usual activities

  ▶ *Call your nurse information service or physician.*

- If you have neck or back pain that does not go away within a few days or is accompanied by fever

  ▶ *Call your nurse information service or physician.*

Treatment

Diagnosing the cause of a back or neck problem can be difficult. Your doctor will take a complete history of the difficulties you are having. He or she will then perform a physical examination to test your range of motion and nerve function. You may also need further tests. These may include X-rays, blood tests, and MRI (magnetic resonance imaging) or CT (computed tomography) scans of your spine.

Most back and neck problems are treated with a combination of rest, medication, and physical therapy. Surgery is not usually recommended, except as a last resort.

Your physician may advise complete bed rest—but probably not for more than one to three days. Lying down for longer periods of time may weaken your muscles and bones and actually slow your recovery. During your rest period, your physician initially may suggest that you apply a cold pack (or a bag of ice) to the painful area for 5 to 10 minutes at a time. The ice will help reduce any inflammation. After about 48 hours you can switch to heat to soothe your symptoms. Try a heating pad or a hot shower or bath. Wearing a soft neck collar (which you can get from your physician) can also help relieve neck pain.

For mild to moderate cases of back or neck pain, an over-the-counter pain reliever, such as acetaminophen, aspirin, ibuprofen, or naproxen, may provide sufficient relief. If your symptoms are severe, your physician may recommend a prescription pain reliever or possibly a muscle relaxant.

You may also be referred to physical therapy treatments. These treatments may include massage, ultrasound, whirlpool baths, and individualized exercise programs to help you regain full use of your back and neck. Spinal manipulation by a licensed chiropractor or other experienced professional may also prove helpful. Some physicians recommend using a *TENS* (*transcutaneous electrical nerve stimulator*). This device relieves pain by sending small electrical impulses through electrodes placed on the skin to underlying nerve fibers.

Remember: Most back and neck problems take time to get better. Feeling a little discomfort as you return to your daily activities is normal, but don't overdo it.

Prevention

- Exercise regularly. It will help keep the muscles that support your back strong and flexible.

- Sleep on a firm mattress.

- To lift a heavy object, bend from the knees, not from the back. Grasp the object and keep it close to your body as you rise. Avoid twisting or bending forward.

- Sit on chairs with good lower back support. Use your arms on the armrests to help lift yourself out of the chair.

- When driving, place a pillow or rolled-up towel behind the small of your back.

- Wear comfortable, low-heeled shoes.

Exercises to Gently Loosen a Stiff Neck

Gently stretch your neck several times a day. It will help keep your neck muscles flexible and strong. *Caution:* Talk to your physician before doing these exercises if you have a neck injury or neck pain.

Stretch #1

1. Keeping your shoulders facing forward, slowly turn your head as far as you can to the right. Hold for 5 seconds. Return your head to center position.

2. Repeat the exercise, turning your head to the left.

3. Do 5 to 10 repetitions of this exercise 3 times a day.

Stretch #2

1. Slowly let your head "drop" toward your right shoulder as though you were trying to touch your right ear to your shoulder. (Be sure to keep your shoulder relaxed.) Hold for 5 seconds. Return your head to center position.

2. Repeat the exercise, tilting your head to your left shoulder.

3. Do 5 to 10 repetitions of this exercise 3 times a day.

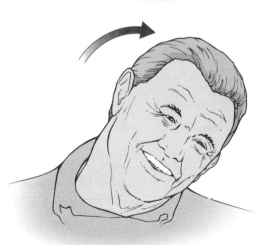

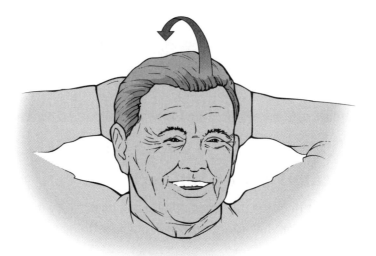

Stretch #3

1. Place both hands behind your head.

2. Try to move your head backward. Use your hands to resist the movement. (Be sure to keep your chin up.) Hold for 5 seconds, then relax.

3. Do 5 to 10 repetitions of this exercise 3 times a day.

Exercise to Gently Stretch Your Lower Back

Stretching your lower back daily can help prevent back pain. *Caution:* Talk to your physician before doing this exercise if you have ever had a back injury.

1. Lie on the floor. Relax your back muscles.

2. Hug your knees to your chest. Pull them in as far as you can without straining. Hold for 15 seconds. (Remember to keep breathing!) Then relax.

3. Do 5 to 10 repetitions of this exercise 3 times a day.

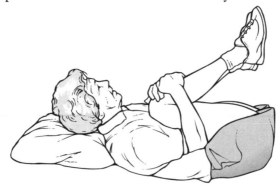

How Will Having a Back or Neck Problem Change My Life?

Having a chronic painful back or neck problem can greatly restrict your movement—and your daily activities. You can't bring in the groceries or swing a grandchild. You may find yourself unable to participate in social situations you used to enjoy. This may lead to anger, frustration, and possibly **depression**, particularly if the pain is intense or chronic. Try to remain as active and involved as possible. Staying active will help you focus your thoughts away from the pain. It will also help you maintain a positive self-image.

Fortunately, most back and neck problems can be cured or managed with proper treatment. If you are experiencing a back or neck problem, don't try to ignore or hide it. See your physician right away. Chances are good that the problem is treatable. You may soon be back to your normal routine, doing the things you like.

But remember: Recovery can be slow. So be patient. Follow your physician's instructions and don't try to force the recovery along too quickly. Also, be clear with family and friends about what you can—and can't—do.

If you feel angry or depressed during the recovery process, you might benefit from talking with a psychologist or other qualified counselor. For a referral, ask your physician. Or call your local mental health organization.

Bladder and Other Urinary Tract Infections

BLADDER and other urinary tract infections (UTIs) are very common. They affect millions of people each year, particularly women. UTIs are usually not serious if caught and treated early. Left untreated, however, they can lead to serious and permanent damage to the kidneys.

Many older people with UTIs often delay getting treatment because they mistakenly blame their symptoms on aging. If you develop any of the symptoms of a UTI, be sure to call your physician right away.

Causes

Some UTIs, particularly in men, are caused by an infection that has migrated to the urinary tract from the prostate gland or some other part of the body. Most UTIs, however, are caused by *E. coli* bacteria. These bacteria are commonly found in the intestines. Sometimes, through poor bathroom hygiene or other habits, the bacteria enter the *urethra*, the tube that carries urine out of the bladder. Once inside the urethra, the bacteria may multiply. They may then move on

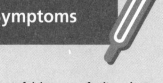

Symptoms

- A painful, burning feeling during urination

- Frequent urge to urinate or **urinary incontinence**

- Blood in the urine

- Milky or cloudy urine

- In women, an uncomfortable pressure around the pubic bone

- In men, a feeling of fullness in the rectum

- Abdominal pain

- Back or side pain

- Fever

- Lethargy

- Mental confusion

When to Seek Help

- If you are having painful urination that is accompanied by fever, bloody urine, vomiting, or abdominal or back pain
  ▶ *Seek emergency care immediately.*

- If you have persistent pain or difficulty urinating
  ▶ *Call your nurse information service or physician.*

- If your urine becomes milky or cloudy
  ▶ *Call your nurse information service or physician.*

- If you become suddenly incontinent
  ▶ *Call your nurse information service or physician.*

to the *bladder*, the chamber in the lower abdomen where urine is stored. If the infection is not stopped, the bacteria may continue to spread up narrow tubes called the *ureters* to the kidneys.

Once the infection reaches the kidneys, it can be life-threatening. The kidneys—a pair of fist-size organs located in your back, just below the bottom ribs on either side of your spine—perform several essential jobs in the body. They remove liquid waste (in the form of urine) from the blood. They make sure that the body's various chemicals stay balanced. And they help regulate blood pressure.

UTIs would be even more common if the urinary tract did not have safeguards that help protect against infection. The flow of urine helps wash bacteria out of the body. And the ureters and bladder usually prevent urine from backing up toward the kidneys. In men, secretions from the prostate gland also help slow down the growth of bacteria.

Women are more at risk than men because their urethra is shorter. This makes it easier for bacteria to travel through the urinary tract. If you are a woman, you have a one in five chance of developing a UTI during your lifetime.

For both men and women, the risk for getting a UTI increases with age. Having **diabetes**, a weakened immune system, kidney stones, or an enlarged prostate gland can also increase your risk. In addition, people who must use *catheters*—tubes inserted into the bladder to empty it—are more likely to experience a UTI.

Sexual activity can also increase the risk for a UTI. An increasing number of UTIs in both men and women have been linked to two sexually transmitted bacteria, *chlamydia* and *mycoplasma*.

Treatment

To find out whether you have a UTI, your physician will usually take a sample of your urine and have it tested for bacteria. UTIs are generally treated with antibiotics. How long you take the antibiotics will depend on the severity of the infection, your age, your general health, and other factors. Be sure to take the antibiotics exactly as instructed by your physician. People who are severely ill with a UTI are sometimes hospitalized until they are able to take enough fluids and medications on their own.

What is...?

...urethritis? An infection limited to the urethra.

...cystitis? An infection of the bladder.

...pyelonephritis? An infection of the kidneys.

If the infection does not get better with treatment, your physician may ask you to come in for special X-ray or ultrasound tests. He or she may also recommend a *cystoscopy*. This test uses a hollow, lighted tube (a *cystoscope*) to examine the inside of the bladder from the urethra.

At-Home Care

- Drink plenty of water—at least 1 to 2 quarts every day.

- Drink cranberry juice every day. It contains substances that keep *E. coli* bacteria from sticking to the lining of the bladder and other parts of the urinary tract. *Caution:* Talk to your physician first. Cranberry juice should not be taken with some medications.

- Empty your bladder as soon as you feel the urge to urinate.

- Avoid spicy foods, alcohol, and all beverages that contain caffeine. They can irritate your bladder.

Prevention

- Follow the tips under "At-Home Care" (opposite).

- Empty your bladder often and completely. Do not hold urine for long periods of time.

- Practice good bathroom hygiene. Thoroughly clean the anal area after a bowel movement. Women should wipe gently from front to back to avoid spreading bacteria from the rectum to the urethra.

- Thoroughly clean the genital area before and after sexual intercourse.

- Empty your bladder after sexual intercourse.

Colds and Flu

THE common cold and the flu (influenza) are often confused with each other. They share similar symptoms: cough, sore throat, and muscle aches and pains. But a cold usually doesn't cause a fever, whereas the flu does. And the flu usually doesn't cause a stuffy nose—a very common symptom of a cold. In general, cold symptoms are milder than those of a flu.

The common cold and the flu are both contagious, spreading easily and quickly from person to person. Both colds and the flu affect millions of Americans each year—and often more than once. In the United States colds tend to strike most often in the fall and winter, the flu in the winter and early spring.

Cold and flu symptoms can differ from person to person. Typical cold symptoms—stuffy nose, sneezing, sore throat, cough—begin two to three days after

Symptoms

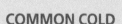

COMMON COLD

- Stuffy nose

- Sneezing

- Itchy or sore throat

- Mild to moderate cough

- Mild muscle aches and fatigue

FLU

- High fever (more than 102 degrees F) that lasts three to four days

- **Headaches** and eye pain

- Severe muscle ache and fatigue

- Extreme exhaustion

- Sore throat

- Dry cough that can become severe

When to Seek Help

- If you experience significant shortness of breath or pain when breathing
  ▶ *Seek emergency care immediately.*

- If you have severe chest pain
  ▶ *Seek emergency care immediately.*

- If you have a temperature of 104 degrees F or higher
  ▶ *Call your nurse information service or physician.*

- If you have cold or flu symptoms and **chronic obstructive pulmonary disease (COPD)**, asthma, or a chronic illness that has compromised your immune system
  ▶ *Call your nurse information service or physician.*

- If you have a severe sore throat and a fever
  ▶ *Call your nurse information service or physician.*

- If your cold does not improve or gets worse after five days
  ▶ *Call your nurse information service or physician.*

- If you have a severe cough with thick yellow-green sputum that may be streaked with blood
  ▶ *Call your nurse information service or physician.*

infection and can last up to 14 days. Flu symptoms—fever, aching muscles, extreme weakness—also start within one to two days of infection and can last up to a week.

Colds and the flu themselves usually are not dangerous. But while your body is fighting off these illnesses, you are at greater risk for developing a second, more serious bacterial infection.

Pneumonia, a severe lung infection, can be a complication of the common cold and especially of the flu. Older people and people with chronic diseases, such as heart problems, asthma, and **cancer**, are at greatest risk for having a cold or the flu develop into **pneumonia**.

Pneumonia can be life-threatening. It is one of the five leading causes of death among people aged 65 and older. That's why it's so important for people in that age group to have an annual flu shot. If you are aged 65 or older, you should also be immunized against pneumococcal **pneumonia**, the type of **pneumonia** that most older people get. You will probably need to get this shot only once. If you haven't had the shot, or are not sure, talk to your physician.

Causes

Colds and the flu are caused by viruses. You can "catch" one of these viruses by breathing in tiny droplets in the air from a sick person's cough or sneeze. You can also become infected by touching something contaminated with the virus—such as a hand, a table, a towel—and then transferring the germs to your nose or eyes.

Cold and flu viruses are constantly mutating, or changing, into new forms. That's why you can never develop a permanent immunity to these illnesses—and why you need to have a new flu shot every year. (There is no vaccine yet for the common cold, mainly because colds are caused by more than 200 different viruses.)

Treatment

Treatment for colds and the flu are similar: Get plenty of rest and drink lots of fluids. For **headaches**, fever, sore throat, and general aches and pains, you may also want to take an over-the-counter pain reliever.

If you have the flu and are at high risk for getting a complication, such as **pneumonia**, your physician may prescribe an antiviral drug, amantadine or rimantidine. Antibiotics are *not* prescribed for colds and the flu. They work only against infections caused by bacteria; they have no effect on viruses.

A Few Words about Over-the-Counter "Cold and Flu" Preparations

Be sure to talk with your physician or pharmacist before taking an over-the-counter preparation for a cold or the flu. These drugs can cause problems for people who have certain health problems, including **coronary heart disease**, **prostate problems**, **diabetes**, **thyroid problems**, and glaucoma. Over-the-counter cold and flu preparations can also interact with other medications you are taking.

Even if you are able to take a cold or flu preparation, you may want to think twice before doing so. In most cases these medications are unnecessary. They may even make your symptoms worse. Here are some tips:

• Avoid "combination" cold and flu preparations—ones that try to treat several symptoms at once. With these medications you'll probably end up treating symptoms you don't have.

• Avoid expectorants. There is no scientific evidence that expectorants actually help loosen mucus.

• Avoid antihistamines. Although helpful for allergies, antihistamines are not generally recommended for colds. Antihistamines can help dry up stuffy nasal passages. But they often thicken the mucus, making it harder to get rid of. Also, in older men antihistamines can lead to urination problems.

• Use cough suppressants sparingly. Cough suppressants can be helpful for a dry, hacking cough. But it's best *not* to suppress a "productive" cough—one that brings mucus up from the lungs. Use suppressants only when a productive cough is so severe that it interferes with sleep or talking.

• Use decongestants sparingly. These medications can help unclog a stuffy nose, but only temporarily. After a few days of use, decongestants often have a "rebound effect." The nasal passages swell up again—sometimes even worse than before.

At-Home Care

- Get plenty of rest.
- Drink plenty of fluids.
- Gargle with warm salt water for a sore throat.
- Use petroleum jelly for a raw nose.
- Take aspirin or acetaminophen for **headaches** or fever.

Prevention

- To avoid picking up viruses, wash your hands often and avoid touching your eyes or nose.
- Get a good night's sleep. If you deprive yourself of sleep, you may weaken your immune system.
- Eat healthful foods (plenty of fruits, vegetables, and whole grains) to keep your immune system strong.
- Don't smoke, and avoid smoky places. Cigarette smokers come down with colds and flus more often than nonsmokers. And the colds and flus they get tend to be more severe.
- Avoid alcohol. Alcohol makes it harder for your body to get rid of cold and flu viruses.
- Exercise daily unless you are ill. Exercise helps keep the immune system strong.
- Avoid close, prolonged exposure to people who have colds.
- Get a flu shot each year. Also, if you are aged 65 or older, be sure you have been immunized against pneumococcal **pneumonia**. You may need the shot sooner if you have had your spleen removed or if you have a chronic disease. Ask your physician.

Constipation

CONSTIPATION is defined as having infrequent bowel movements or having hard, dry stools that are difficult or painful to pass. Everyone gets constipated from time to time. The problem is usually short-lived and easily corrected with a simple change in diet.

Sometimes, however, the problem may develop into *fecal impaction*, a severe form of constipation in which a large mass of stool cannot be passed. When this happens, you may need to see your physician to have the stool removed manually or by a mild enema.

Many people think they are constipated when they are not. They mistakenly believe that everyone should have at least one bowel movement every day. Actually, the frequency of bowel movements in healthy people can vary from three a day to three a week. Some people can go as long as a week between bowel movements without any discomfort or harmful effect.

Constipation often causes people to strain when having a bowel movement. This straining can lead to complications such as **hemorrhoids** (swollen and painful veins around the anus and lower rectum) and fissures (small tears in the lining of the anus that cause pain, bleeding, and itching). It also can be associated with **diverticulitis**, a serious inflammation of the colon. In rare cases straining causes a small amount of intestinal lining to push out from the rectal opening. This condition is known as *rectal prolapse*.

Constipation can also be a symptom of a more serious underlying disorder or disease. If your constipation is severe or continues for more than two weeks, call your physician.

Symptoms

- Infrequent bowel movements (fewer than three a week)

- Hard, dry stools that are sometimes painful to pass

When to Seek Help

- If you have blood in your stool ▶ *Call your nurse information service or physician.*

- If your constipation is accompanied by fever and abdominal pain ▶ *Call your nurse information service or physician.*

- If you are constipated for more than two weeks ▶ *Call your nurse information service or physician.*

- If your constipation begins after starting a new medication or vitamin or mineral supplement ▶ *Call your nurse information service or physician.*

- If you experience a significant and prolonged change of bowel habits ▶ *Call your nurse information service or physician.*

Causes

Not eating enough fiber, not drinking enough fluids, and not exercising regularly are among the most common causes of constipation. Certain medications and vitamin and mineral supplements can also cause stools to become hardened and difficult to pass. Let your physician know if you become constipated after starting a new medication.

Repeatedly ignoring the urge to have a bowel movement can also lead to constipation. So can misusing laxatives (see "Laxatives: Break the Habit," p. 134).

Disorders and diseases that can cause constipation include irritable bowel syndrome, **thyroid problems**, colorectal **cancer**, **diabetes**, **Parkinson's disease**, and **depression**.

Treatment

Most cases of constipation respond to simple changes in diet. Eat more fiber-rich foods, such as unprocessed bran, whole-grain bread, and fresh fruits and vegetables. Nutrition experts recommend you try to eat at least 30 grams of fiber each day. Most people eat only about 12 to 15 grams of fiber per day. (For a listing of foods and their fiber content, see p. 10.) Add the fiber to your diet gradually. This will give your digestive system time to adapt. And drink plenty of water—at least eight glasses a day.

If you develop fecal impaction, your physician may recommend an enema. Your physician may also break up the hardened stool manually by inserting a gloved finger into the rectum.

At-Home Care

- Eat more high-fiber foods—fresh fruits and vegetables, whole-wheat grains, and unprocessed bran.

- Drink plenty of liquids—at least eight glasses a day.

- Get moving. Exercise helps stimulate activity in the bowels.

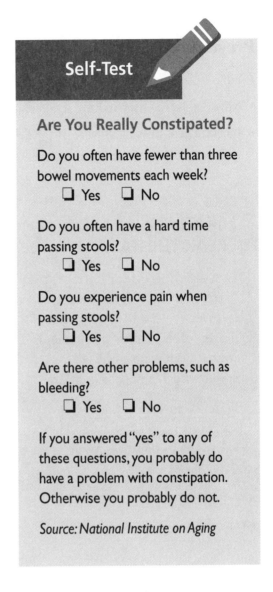

Self-Test

Are You Really Constipated?

Do you often have fewer than three bowel movements each week?
❏ Yes   ❏ No

Do you often have a hard time passing stools?
❏ Yes   ❏ No

Do you experience pain when passing stools?
❏ Yes   ❏ No

Are there other problems, such as bleeding?
❏ Yes   ❏ No

If you answered "yes" to any of these questions, you probably do have a problem with constipation. Otherwise you probably do not.

Source: National Institute on Aging

Prevention

- Follow the tips under "At-Home Care" (p. 133).

- Never resist the urge to have a bowel movement.

- Use laxatives only as a last resort. Never use them for more than a few days at any one time. Remember: It is not necessary to have a bowel movement every day.

LAXATIVES: BREAK THE HABIT

Each year Americans spend more than $700 million on over-the-counter laxatives—medications designed to loosen stools. Much of that money is wasted. Most people who are constipated do not need laxatives.

In fact, laxative use is one of the leading *causes* of constipation. Here's why: If you use laxatives regularly, your body may become dependent on them. You will then need to take increasing amounts of the laxatives to keep from becoming constipated.

Health experts recommend taking laxatives only as a last resort, after all other self-help efforts have failed. They also should be taken only under the supervision of a physician. If you have been using laxatives for a long time, talk to your physician about how you should discontinue their use.

Foot Complaints

OUR feet change as we grow older. Our toenails get thicker and more brittle. Our skin becomes drier. The pads that cushion the bottom of our feet become thinner and less protective. As we age, we also tend to put on weight, which adds extra stress to the bones and ligaments of our feet. In addition, our feet tend to spread—although we often continue to cram them into the same old shoe size.

Foot ailments come in many different forms—more than 300 in all. Some are inherited, but most are the result of years of neglect or abuse. We often don't think about taking care of our feet until they begin to cause us pain or discomfort.

Symptoms

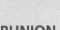

BUNION

- An enlargement at the joint of the big or small toe (bunionette)

- Swelling, redness, and pain at the joint of the big or small toe

HAMMERTOE

- A toe (usually the second toe) that bends up permanently at the middle joint

HEEL PAIN

- Pain either below or behind the heel of the foot

INGROWN TOENAIL

- Pain and redness around a toenail, especially the nail of the big toe

CORN OR CALLUS

- A patch of thickened, dead skin on the top of the toes (corn) or the bottom of the foot (callus)

MORTON'S NEUROMA

- Pain, numbness, or a tingling sensation between the toes and in the ball of the foot

When to Seek Help

- If a foot or toe becomes suddenly cold, numb, or blue ▶ *Seek emergency care immediately.*

- If you are experiencing pain in your foot that persists or becomes disabling ▶ *Call your nurse information service or physician.*

- If an ingrown toenail, a corn, or a callus becomes infected or another area of the affected foot appears reddened or feels hot ▶ *Call your nurse information service or physician.*

- If you have a burning or tingling sensation in your feet ▶ *Call your nurse information service or physician.*

- If your feet appear discolored ▶ *Call your nurse information service or physician.*

Foot problems frequently keep older people from leading active lives. They can also lead to knee, hip, and lower back pain, which can further limit our ability to move around. Fortunately, many foot problems can be treated successfully. As with any condition or illness, it's important to catch the problem early.

Bunions

A bunion is a painful enlargement at the joint of the big toe. Sometimes the swelling pushes the big toe inward, making it overlap one or more of the other toes. A similar condition—called a *bunionette* or *tailor's bunion*—can also develop on the little toe.

Causes

Some people get bunions because of years of wearing tight, poorly fitting shoes. Heredity, however, is the main reason people get bunions. People with low arches ("flat feet"), for example, are more likely to develop the problem than people with higher arches. Bunions have also been linked to **arthritis** in older people.

Treatment

Wear well-made shoes that fit properly. Avoid shoes that cramp or pinch your toes. To relieve the immediate pain of a bunion, try an over-the-counter pain reliever. You can also try soaking your foot in warm water or applying a heating pad to the swollen joint. Bunion pads, which you can buy at a drugstore, can offer some relief. Stop using the pads, however, if they start exerting pressure elsewhere on your foot.

If the pain persists or if the bunion interferes with your ability to walk comfortably, see your physician or a *podiatrist* (a physician who specializes in disorders of the feet). You may be prescribed special shoe inserts called *orthotics* to help take some of the pressure off your swollen joint. Cortisone injections may also be prescribed. In severe cases surgery is sometimes recommended to help realign the big toe and relieve the pain.

Hammertoe

A hammertoe is a foot deformity in which the tendons or ligaments in a toe become stretched or tightened, causing the toe to bend up permanently at the middle joint. The second toe is most likely to develop into a hammertoe, but any of the other three smaller toes can also be affected.

Often a foot with a hammertoe will also have a bunion. The bunion pushes the big toe under the second toe, buckling it. The tops of hammertoes can rub against shoes, causing painful corns and calluses to form.

Causes

Hammertoes are often inherited. People with high arches, rheumatoid **arthritis**, or feet that *pronate* (roll inward when walking) are especially susceptible to developing hammertoes. Wearing shoes that are too tight or too small can make the problem worse.

Treatment

Wear shoes and socks that have plenty of toe room. If the pain persists, see your physician or a podiatrist. Surgery is sometimes recommended in advanced cases.

Heel Pain

Heel pain happens when the tissues, nerves, or bone of the heel become irritated or inflamed. The condition is sometimes linked to *plantar fasciitis,* an inflammation of the long band of connective tissue that runs along the sole of the foot. Heel pain is also associated with *spurs*—calcium growths that can develop on the bones of the feet.

> ### A CHECKLIST FOR SHOES
>
> - **Good fit**—comfortably loose when worn with soft, absorbent socks.
>
> - **Shaped like the foot**—broad and spacious in the toe area.
>
> - **Shock-absorbent sole**—a low-wedge type is best; avoid high heels.
>
> - **Breathable material**—canvas or leather, not plastic.
>
> - **Comfortable**—the moment you put them on.
>
> *Source: American Orthopaedic Foot and Ankle Society*

Causes

Heel pain usually occurs when too much stress is put on the feet. Walking or standing on hard surfaces for long periods of time can cause the pain, especially when wearing poorly made shoes. **Arthritis**, circulatory problems, and other health conditions can also lead to heel pain. And being overweight can aggravate the condition.

Treatment

Try different shoes, and rest your feet whenever possible. Heel pain often improves spontaneously. If the pain persists, however, see your physician or a podiatrist. Your physician may recommend special stretching exercises and shoe inserts. Sometimes cortisone injections are prescribed. Surgery is rarely necessary.

Ingrown Toenails

Ingrown toenails are nails that grow into the skin instead of over it. The skin around the toenail may become red and infected. The big toes are most often affected, but any toenail can become ingrown.

Causes

Ingrown toenails are usually the result of trimming nails too short, particularly at the sides. But tight shoes or stockings, a foot injury, a fungus infection, or poor foot structure can also contribute to the problem.

Treatment

To treat an ingrown toenail, soften the nail by soaking your foot in warm salt water. Gently slip a piece of sterile cotton with an over-the-counter antibiotic ointment under the corner of the nail. Change the cotton daily. (*Caution:* If you have **diabetes** or a circulatory problem, be sure to seek medical attention for your ingrown toenail before treating it yourself.) If the pain does not go away after a few days or the nail becomes infected (pus develops), call your physician. In severe cases the nail may be partially or completely removed.

Most ingrown toenails can be prevented with proper foot care. Trim your toenails straight across. The nails should be level with, or slightly longer than, the top of the toe. If you have difficulty trimming your own nails, talk to your physician about having them done during your regular medical checkups.

Corns and Calluses

A corn is a thickening of the skin, usually on the top of the toes. A callus is the same condition, but on the bottom of the feet. Both corns and calluses can become infected through a break in the skin.

Should a corn or callus become infected, call your physician or a podiatrist. Oral antibiotics are sometimes prescribed for infected corns and calluses.

Causes

Most corns and calluses are caused by friction or pressure on the skin of the foot. Poorly fitting shoes are usually the culprit. In some cases calluses appear where there is no apparent friction or pressure. These are known as *hereditary calluses* and tend to run in families.

Treatment

Most corns and calluses go away once the source of the friction or pressure is removed. Your best treatment, therefore, is to wear properly fitting shoes. Avoid pointed shoes and high heels. Over-the-counter salicylic-acid corn remedies and corn plasters are generally not recommended. They can destroy healthy skin around the corn.

To help remove a corn or callus, soak your feet in an Epsom salts footbath every day. You can use a pumice or callus file to gently rub dead skin off a callus. Do not rub corns; it may make them more tender and painful. Also, *never* cut a corn or a callus to remove the skin; cutting can lead to an infection. *Caution:* Do not attempt these home treatments if you have **diabetes** or a circulatory problem. Talk to your physician first.

CAUTION

A SPECIAL WARNING FOR PEOPLE WITH DIABETES

Diabetes can damage nerves, making it difficult to perceive pain. A small problem, such as an ingrown toenail, may develop into a big infection before you notice that anything is wrong.

If you have **diabetes**, you need to take special care of your feet. Wear comfortable shoes and bathe your feet every day. You should also inspect your feet daily. Be sure to report any redness, cuts, blisters, swelling, or sign of infection to your physician right away.

Morton's Neuroma

A Morton's neuroma is a thickening of nerve tissue, usually between the third and fourth toes. The neuroma can cause pain, numbness, or a tingling sensation between the toes and in the ball of the foot.

Causes

Although the exact cause of neuromas is unknown, doctors believe the condition develops when two bones in the foot rub and "pinch" a nerve. The nerve then becomes inflamed and thickens. The problem can be triggered by an abnormal bone structure, an injury, or ill-fitting shoes.

Treatment

Early treatment can help you avoid surgery later. You should seek medical care for a neuroma as soon as the symptoms develop. Your physician or podiatrist may recommend special stretching exercises and shoe inserts. You'll also be advised to wear shoes with wide toeboxes. Sometimes cortisone injections are prescribed. If the problem continues, surgery to remove the neuroma may be an option.

Prevention

- Wear low-heeled, roomy, well-cushioned shoes.
- Always have your feet measured before buying new shoes.
- Make sure your pantyhose or stockings are not too tight.
- Never cut corns or calluses.
- Bathe your feet daily in lukewarm water.
- Trim your toenails straight across.
- Inspect your feet regularly, or have someone do this for you.

Gallstones

THE gallbladder is a pear-shaped organ located underneath the liver in the upper right abdomen. It stores *bile*, a liquid that helps the body digest fats. Bile travels from the gallbladder to the small intestine through tubes called *ducts*.

Sometimes the bile in the gallbladder or ducts hardens into small lumps. These are known as *gallbladder stones*, or *gallstones*. The stones can be as small as a grain of sand or as big as a golf ball.

Most gallstones cause no discomfort and require no treatment. Sometimes, however, a stone gets trapped in one of the bile ducts. This can cause a painful gallstone "attack"—several hours of pain, nausea, gas, and **indigestion**—before the stone dissolves or becomes dislodged. If the blockage continues, it can eventually cause severe—even life-threatening—damage to the gallbladder, liver, or pancreas. You should call your physician immediately if you are experiencing symptoms of a gallbladder attack.

Causes

Gallstones form when your bile becomes chemically imbalanced. The people who are at greatest risk for developing this bile imbalance—and gallstones—include the following:

- People over age 60
- Women
- Native Americans
- Mexican Americans

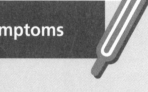

Symptoms

- Steady, severe pain in the upper abdomen that increases rapidly and lasts from 30 minutes to several hours; pain may extend to the back, chest, or right shoulder

- Nausea or vomiting

- Gas and **indigestion**

- Fever and chills

- Yellowish skin and eyes (jaundice)

- Tea- or coffee-colored urine

When to Seek Help

- If you are experiencing steady, severe pain in your upper abdomen that radiates to your back, chest, or shoulders ► *Seek emergency care immediately.*

- If you are experiencing other symptoms of gallstones (opposite) ► *Call your nurse information service or physician.*

- Overweight men and women
- People who fast or lose a lot of weight quickly
- Women on hormone replacement therapy
- People taking cholesterol-lowering drugs
- People with **diabetes**

Treatment

Your physician may use several tests to determine whether your symptoms are caused by gallstones. Your blood will be tested for signs of infection and obstruction. You may also undergo an *ultrasound* exam. An ultrasound uses sound waves to create pictures of the gallbladder and bile ducts. You may also be given other, more complicated tests. One of these tests goes by the acronym *ERCP (endoscopic retrograde cholangiopancreatography)*. It uses an *endoscope*, a long, flexible, lighted tube connected to a computer and TV monitor. The tube is slipped down the patient's throat and guided into the small intestine. Once in place, it can help locate gallstones in the bile ducts.

Surgery is the most common treatment for gallstones that are causing symptoms. The surgery—called a *cholecystectomy*—removes the gallbladder. In years past, all gallbladders were removed with "open" abdominal surgery. Today, most gallbladder surgery is done using a *laparoscope*, a thin, lighted tube that is inserted into the abdomen through a tiny incision. The smaller incision usually means less pain after the operation. It also means shorter hospital stays, less scarring, and a quicker return to normal activity.

Fortunately, people can live quite well without their gallbladder. Not having a gallbladder does cause diarrhea in some people, however. It may also cause higher blood cholesterol levels. People who have had their gallbladder removed should be sure to have their cholesterol checked regularly.

Sometimes health problems or other special circumstances make gallbladder surgery inadvisable. Nonsurgical treatments such as drugs and shock wave therapy may be recommended; both are designed to break up existing stones. However, nonsurgical treatments often have serious side effects and are effective only about half the time. They also do not keep new stones from forming.

Prevention

- Maintain a normal weight.
- Avoid crash diets.
- Exercise regularly.

Hair Loss

MOST people experience some kind of hair loss during their lives. That's because our hair thins naturally as we grow older. Excessive thinning of hair can lead to baldness, or *alopecia*. About 40 million men and 20 million women in the United States have some amount of balding.

Men and women tend to lose hair differently. Men can start going bald in their late teens or early 20s. Women usually don't experience a significant thinning of their hair until their 40s or later. Men and women also tend to have different patterns of balding (see p. 147).

Causes

Most hair loss is hereditary. The genes for hair loss are passed down through both parents (not just through the father, as commonly believed). Several conditions and illnesses can also cause hair to fall out, but usually for only a short time. These include the following:

- High fever
- **Thyroid problems**
- Physical and emotional stress
- Certain medications, including drugs used to treat **arthritis**, **depression**, heart problems, **high blood pressure**, or **cancer**
- Severe lack of protein in the diet
- Severe lack of iron in the diet
- Major surgery or a severe chronic illness

Symptoms

- Thinning or loss of hair on scalp
- Receding hairline
- Complete loss of all hair on the body
- Excessive shedding of hair

Damage can cause hair to thin. Common sources of hair damage include improper or too frequent use of bleaches, dyes, straighteners, hair weaving, permanent waves, hair dryers, and hot curlers.

Treatment

Many people live quite contentedly with naturally thinning hair or balding hairlines. They are comfortable with their appearance and feel no need to replace lost hair.

When to Seek Help

• If you experience any sudden, unexplained hair loss

Call your nurse information service or physician.

Some people find that special kinds of haircuts and cosmetic techniques, such as permanent waves, can help disguise thinning hair. Others opt for hair additions—such as wigs, hairpieces, and hair weaving—to cover bald areas.

The Food and Drug Administration (FDA) has approved two medications for regrowing hair. The drug minoxidil has been shown to be effective in slowing hair loss in some men and women. It is applied topically to balding spots twice a day. Minoxidil is available over the counter and in stronger concentrations with a doctor's prescription. *Caution:* If you have any kind of heart disease, you should talk to your physician before using this drug.

Another drug, finasteride, has also been approved by the FDA for regrowing hair, but in men only. It is available only by prescription.

Hair replacement surgery is sometimes an option for people who have experienced permanent hair loss. In transplantation surgery, plugs of skin containing active hair follicles are transplanted from densely covered areas of the head to balding spots. Another type of surgery, scalp reduction, involves removing sections of bald scalp. Areas of the scalp that do contain hair are then pulled toward the crown.

If your hair loss is health related, your physician will treat the underlying condition. If your hair loss is due to a particular medication, your physician may switch you to a different one.

HOW MEN LOSE THEIR HAIR

Men tend to lose their hair from the forehead and temple and then from the crown (left). Often, what is left is a horseshoe-shaped fringe of hair around the sides and back of the head (right).

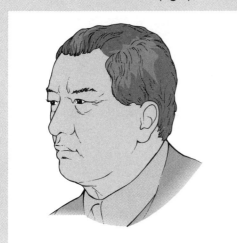
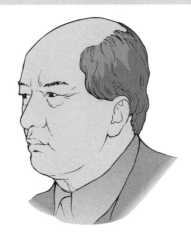

HOW WOMEN LOSE THEIR HAIR

The thinning of women's hair tends to start at the crown (left). In a small percentage of women, the crown may become almost completely bald (right).

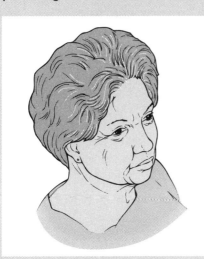
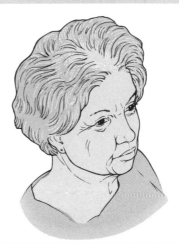

Prevention

- Protect your hair from damage (such as overuse of bleaches, dyes, and hair dryers) that may eventually lead to thinning.

- To prevent diet-related hair loss, eat a well-balanced diet.

How Will Losing My Hair Change My Life?

Losing your hair needn't change your life at all. Unless related to an illness, hair loss has no effect on physical health. One of the biggest myths about hair loss is that it affects virility. It does not.

Losing one's hair can be an emotional experience, however. It can lead to **anxiety**, irritation, **grief**, and **depression**. Self-esteem can plummet as people mistakenly believe they are no longer "attractive." But remember: There is no single standard of attractiveness. (Just think of Yul Brynner!) Your attitude toward life plays a much bigger role in your personal "appeal."

If your hair loss is filling you with feelings of self-consciousness, **anxiety**, or **depression**, then you may benefit from talking with a psychologist or other qualified counselor about your concerns. If your hair loss is the result of an illness, consider joining a support group for people who are going through a similar experience. Your physician can help you find such a group near you.

Did You Know?

The average person has about 100,000 scalp hairs. About 50 to 100 of these hairs are shed each day. So finding a few hairs on your hairbrush or comb is not necessarily a sign that you are going bald!

Headaches

ALMOST everyone gets headaches from time to time. Most headaches are mild and harmless and vanish once you've taken aspirin or another pain reliever. Others are more severe and sometimes incapacitating while they last. Headaches can be short-lived or chronic, striking repeatedly for many years. Chronic headaches are particularly common among older people; about half of people over the age of 60 report having frequent mild to severe headaches.

There are four main types of headaches: tension, migraine, cluster, and sinus. About 90 percent of headaches are *tension headaches*—a dull, steady pressure in the head that worsens as the day goes on. These headaches may come with muscle tightness in the neck, back, and shoulders.

A *migraine headache* typically causes intense, throbbing pain. It often starts on one side of the head or behind the eyes. Some people feel nauseated or see flashing lights or spots (called an *aura*) just before the headache strikes. A migraine can last from a few hours to a few days. These headaches are more common in women than in men and tend to run in families.

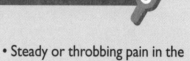

Symptoms

- Steady or throbbing pain in the head or inside of the face

- Sometimes nausea or dizziness

The sharp, often excruciating pain of a *cluster headache* usually starts behind one eye and spreads to that side of the head. The eye may become red and watery. A cluster headache can last from 15 minutes to several hours. They come and go in "clusters" over a period of days or weeks, then mysteriously disappear for months or years. Cluster headaches are more common in men than in women.

A *sinus headache* is characterized by pain and pressure in or around the eyes or forehead. The pain may also spread to the top of the head and may worsen when

When to Seek Help

- If your headache is sudden or severe (the worst you have experienced in your life) and comes with symptoms such as nausea, vomiting, **vision problems**, slurred speech, or tingling or numbness in a part of your body

  ▶ *Seek emergency care immediately.*

- If your headache is severe and comes with high fever, nausea, stiff neck, drowsiness, and an inability to tolerate bright light

  ▶ *Seek emergency care immediately.*

- If your headache follows a head injury

  ▶ *Seek emergency care immediately.*

- If your headache lasts longer than 24 hours

  ▶ *Call your nurse information service or physician.*

- If your headache is chronic (returns as often as once a week)

  ▶ *Call your nurse information service or physician.*

you lean forward. Sinus headaches often come with other symptoms, such as a runny nose, watery eyes, and sneezing.

Causes

Headaches have many causes. Tension headaches strike when muscles become tight, usually because of stress or poor posture. Other common causes of tension headaches include eyestrain and grinding or clenching teeth while sleeping.

Migraine headaches begin when blood vessels in the brain narrow and then widen. This swelling seems to stimulate nerves in the head. Many things can trigger a migraine, including stress, caffeine, certain foods, or odors—even a change in weather. In some women, declining levels of the hormone estrogen after **menopause** can also lead to migraines.

Cluster headaches are also caused by changes in the flow of blood to the head. Just what triggers those changes is not entirely clear. But people who smoke heavily or who drink a lot of alcohol are more likely to get cluster headaches.

Sinus headaches are usually the result of allergies, colds, or the flu.

A severe headache is sometimes a sign of a serious health problem, such as **stroke** or meningitis, a life-threatening infection of the membranes covering the spinal cord and brain. Tension headaches can be a sign of **depression**, particularly in older people.

Treatment

Most tension headaches can be relieved with rest and an over-the-counter pain reliever. Sinus headaches are often treated with decongestants. If your headache is the result of a sinus infection, you may be given antibiotics.

The pain of a migraine headache can sometimes be stopped or reduced by sleep and/or by taking an over-the-counter pain reliever right when the headache begins. In most cases, however, prescription drugs are needed.

If you suffer from frequent migraine or cluster headaches, see your physician. Your physician can prescribe medications to both relieve and prevent chronic headaches. To relieve cluster headaches, your physician may recommend that you inhale pure oxygen from a tank that you can purchase and keep in your home.

At-Home Care

- At the first sign of a headache, lie down in a dark, quiet room. Try to sleep.

- Take an over-the-counter pain reliever.

- Apply an ice pack or cold compress to your head.

- Gently massage your forehead and temples.

Prevention

- Keep a headache "diary." Write down when each headache strikes and what you were doing or eating in the hours before. Keeping track of headaches can help you avoid triggers.

- If you get migraines, avoid foods that contain the substance tyramine, which is known to trigger headaches in some people. Such foods include aged cheeses, pickled herring, red wine, beer, liver, pizza, fava beans, and peanut butter.

CAUTION

Avoid taking over-the-counter pain medications, especially those containing caffeine, more often than three times a week. If taken too frequently, these drugs can have a rebound effect. They may eventually make your headaches worse.

- Avoid oversleeping on weekends. Sleeping late can cause your body's normal blood sugar level to drop, leading to a headache.

- If you grind your teeth at night, try wearing a bite guard while you sleep. Ask your dentist for advice on what kind of bite guard to purchase.

- Reduce stress by exercising, stretching, and taking rest breaks.

Hearing Problems

HEARING loss is common among older people. About one-third of Americans between the ages of 65 and 74 and about one-half of those aged 85 and older have a hearing problem. Such problems can be minor, such as missing certain high-pitched sounds, or serious, resulting in total deafness.

The most common type of age-related hearing loss is known as *presbycusis*. It usually begins between the ages of 40 and 50 and then slowly worsens. People with presbycusis have a difficult time hearing what others are saying—particularly the high-pitched voices of women and children. They may also be unable to tolerate loud sounds. Presbycusis tends to affect men more than women. Because the hearing loss is gradual, people with presbycusis may not be aware that they are experiencing it until it becomes very noticeable.

Another common hearing problem in older people is *tinnitus*. People with this disorder hear a ringing, roaring, buzzing, hissing, or other sound inside the ears. The sound can vary in loudness and may be constant or come and go. It tends to be loudest when background noise is low, such as when trying to fall asleep. People with tinnitus may not necessarily have a hearing loss. In fact, many people with tinnitus are extremely sensitive to noise.

Causes

Some types of hearing loss— known as *conductive hearing loss*— happen when something blocks

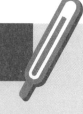

Symptoms

- Difficulty distinguishing some or all sounds in one or both ears

- Difficulty understanding another person's speech, especially when there is background noise

- Sensitivity to certain sounds, which seem overly loud or annoying

- Difficulty hearing the TV or radio unless the volume is turned up high

- Ringing or hissing sound in the ears

When to Seek Help

• If you are having some hearing loss and pus, fluid, or blood is draining from your ear	▶ *Call your nurse information service or physician immediately.*
• If you are having any hearing problems	▶ *Call your nurse information service or physician.*
• If you have a sudden and total hearing loss in one or both ears	▶ *Call your nurse information service or physician.*
• If your hearing loss is accompanied by dizziness or nausea	▶ *Call your nurse information service or physician.*

sound waves from traveling from the outer to the inner ear. The most common reasons for these blockages are excessive earwax and ear infections, although sometimes a benign cyst, a tumor, or a trapped insect can create a "sound barrier" within the ear.

Sensorineural hearing loss happens when parts of the inner ear or the auditory nerve (the nerve that sends sound impulses from the inner ear to the brain) become damaged. This type of hearing loss can be caused by birth defects, head injury, tumors, illness, certain medications (including some types of antibiotics, diuretics, and high doses of aspirin), poor blood circulation, **high blood pressure**, or **stroke**. It can also result from prolonged exposure to loud noises. People who work at a particularly noisy job, such as carpentry or street repair work, or who have noisy hobbies, such as hunting, snowmobiling, or listening to loud, amplified music, particularly with headphones, are at increased risk for developing a permanent hearing loss.

Presbycusis is usually a sensorineural hearing disorder. In most cases it is the result of a loss of hair cells within the inner ear. The cells are needed to help transfer sound vibrations into the nerve signals that travel to the brain. Various health conditions, such as **coronary heart disease**, **high blood pressure**, and **diabetes**, can cause the hair cells to be destroyed, as can certain medications and exposure to loud sounds. Genetics also plays a major role in the development of presbycusis: This type of hearing loss tends to run in families.

Causes of tinnitus include excessive earwax, ear infections, tumors, a perforated eardrum, and certain medications, including aspirin. But the most common cause is exposure to loud noise, either over a long period of time or during one extreme incident.

Diagnosis and Treatment

If you are having trouble hearing, see your physician. He or she will carefully examine your ears and perhaps give you a few simple hearing tests. If your physician cannot identify the source of the problem, you may be referred to an *otolaryngologist.* This physician specializes in treatments of the ear, nose, and throat. You may also be referred to an *audiologist,* a nonphysician health professional who can identify and measure hearing loss. Using a device called an *audiometer,* the audiologist will test your ability to hear sounds at various pitches and loudness. The test is painless.

The treatment for hearing loss depends upon its cause. If you have a temporary hearing loss due to excessive earwax, your physician will clean out your ears, perhaps with a suction device. If you have an ear infection or a ruptured

IF SOMEONE YOU KNOW HAS A HEARING PROBLEM

- Face the person and talk clearly.

- Stand where there is good lighting and low background noise.

- Speak clearly and at a reasonable speed; do not hide your mouth, eat, or chew gum while speaking.

- Use facial expressions or gestures to give useful clues.

- Reword your statement if needed.

- Be patient, stay positive and relaxed.

- Ask how you may help the listener.

- Include the person with a hearing impairment in all discussions about him or her to prevent feelings of isolation.

Source: National Institute on Aging

eardrum, your physician will probably prescribe antibiotics. In some rare cases minor surgery is required to repair a ruptured eardrum.

No medications or surgery can reverse a permanent hearing loss, such as presbycusis. The only method of treatment for presbycusis is a hearing aid, a small device that fits in the ear and helps make sounds louder. Hearing aids are also sometimes helpful for people with tinnitus. Treatment options for tinnitus include medication, masking (covering up the unwanted sound with a more pleasant one), and biofeedback.

Living with a Hearing Problem

TIPS ON BUYING A HEARING AID

You should see a physician for a medical evaluation before you buy a hearing aid. If you do not receive a medical evaluation, you will be required to sign a waiver saying that you did not want the exam before purchasing the hearing aid.

You can be fitted for a hearing aid by an otolaryngologist, audiologist, or independent dispenser. Your hearing aid should be custom fitted to your ear and hearing needs. Remember: You are buying a service as well as a product. Most hearing aids require some fitting adjustments. Be sure the person you are purchasing the hearing aid from has the patience and skill to help you during the month or so it takes to adjust to the new device.

- Tell others that you have trouble hearing. Ask them to face you, to speak more slowly and clearly, and not to shout.

- Pay close attention when people are talking. Watch facial expressions and gestures to better understand what is being said.

- Tell people when you have trouble understanding them. Ask them to repeat what they said.

- Use assistive listening devices, such as a telephone amplifier.

- If you have tinnitus, avoid alcohol, smoking, caffeine, and large doses of aspirin, which can make the condition worse.

- When dining out, choose less noisy restaurants and try to be seated against the wall, not in the middle of the room.

Prevention

- Avoid loud sounds. If you must be exposed to harmful levels of noise, protect your ears by wearing earplugs. *Caution:* Do not use cottonballs as earplugs. They will not protect your ears from loud sounds and may get lodged in your ear canal.

- Never listen to loud music with earphones.

How Will Having a Hearing Loss Change My Life?

An unrecognized hearing loss can have a profound effect on your life. Unable to hear clearly, you may begin to misinterpret conversations. You may start to grumble that people are "mumbling" or "garbling their words," not realizing that high-pitched voices—particularly those of children—are hard to hear.

Your hearing loss may begin to affect your relationships with your friends and family. They may start to raise their voices. Or they may find they need to repeat what they say to you several times. Having to "shout" can be stressful. People may become reluctant to start a conversation with you. As you find it more difficult to communicate, you may become distrustful, depressed, or withdrawn. You may find yourself avoiding social situations you used to enjoy, such as concerts, club meetings, and dining out.

Fortunately, most permanent hearing losses can be corrected with a hearing aid. Yet only about one in five people who would benefit from a hearing aid actually use one. If you have a hearing problem, see your physician. You can get help.

Hemorrhoids

HEMORRHOIDS are swollen blood vessels in and around the anus and lower rectum. They are also known as *piles* or sometimes as "the **varicose veins** of the rectum." Although hemorrhoids can be quite painful, they are usually harmless and go away within a few days. They are a very common ailment: More than half of the people in the United States have hemorrhoids by the time they are 50 years old.

Hemorrhoids develop either under the skin around the anus (external) or inside the anus (internal). An external hemorrhoid feels like a hard, painful lump. It bleeds only when it is ruptured. An internal hemorrhoid is often painless. Bleeding may be the only sign of its existence. Sometimes internal hemorrhoids *prolapse*, or enlarge, and protrude from the anal opening. A prolapsed hemorrhoid can cause severe pain.

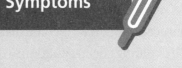

Symptoms

- Bleeding during bowel movements
- Tenderness or pain during bowel movements
- Itching in the anal area
- Painful swelling or hard lump around the anus
- A discharge of mucus from the anus

Causes

The exact cause of hemorrhoids is not known. They often are a result, however, of straining during bowel movements. Chronic **constipation**, therefore, can lead to hemorrhoids. So can chronic diarrhea and an overuse of laxatives. Aging and heredity also appear to play a role in the development of hemorrhoids.

Treatment

Most hemorrhoids can be treated with at-home care, such as ice packs and warm baths. If you experience severe, persistent pain, your physician may

When to Seek Help

- If you experience any amount of new anal bleeding ▶ **Call your nurse information service or physician.**

- If pain from the hemorrhoids is lasting or severe ▶ **Call your nurse information service or physician.**

recommend that the hemorrhoid be removed. Several methods, ranging from chemical injections to surgery, are used to remove hemorrhoids.

At-Home Care

- Try an over-the-counter stool softener if bowel movements have been hard.

- Take a warm tub bath several times a day. Pat dry gently.

- Use ice packs to help reduce swelling and itching.

- Dab witch hazel gently on the outside of the anus to help reduce pain and itching.

- Place some petroleum jelly inside and around the edge of the anus to make bowel movements less painful. When wiping the anus after a bowel movement, special wipes made for hemorrhoids or cotton pads soaked in witch hazel can be soothing.

- Avoid scratching hemorrhoids.

Prevention

- Eat a high-fiber diet—plenty of fruits, vegetables, and whole-grain breads and cereals.

- Eat less meat and animal fat, and drink less alcohol.

- Avoid sitting for long periods. Get up and walk around. Sitting for long periods of time reduces blood flow around the anus.

- Exercise regularly. It can help you avoid **constipation**.

Indigestion and Heartburn

INDIGESTION is a painful burning sensation in the upper abdomen. It is also known as *upset stomach* or *dyspepsia*. Often it is accompanied by nausea, abdominal bloating, belching, or, rarely, vomiting. Indigestion is sometimes a symptom of an underlying disease or disorder, such as **gallstones**.

Heartburn, also called *acid indigestion* or *gastroesophageal reflux disease*, is a burning feeling right behind the breastbone. But it has nothing to do with the heart. Heartburn results from stomach acids backing up into the lower esophagus (the tube that leads from the throat to the stomach). About 1 in 10 adults has heartburn at least once a week, and 1 in 3 has it monthly.

Causes

Indigestion has many causes. Sometimes it is the result of a **stomach ulcer** or a disease in the digestive tract. But often indigestion is caused by poor eating habits. People who overeat or who eat too quickly or while under stress are more likely to suffer from indigestion. Other common causes of indigestion include smoking, eating high-fat foods, drinking too much alcohol, and using medications, such as aspirin, that irritate the stomach lining. Obesity can also lead to chronic indigestion.

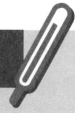

Symptoms

INDIGESTION

- Abdominal bloating and/or pain
- Gas or belching
- Mild nausea

HEARTBURN

- Burning chest pain that begins behind the breastbone and moves upward to the neck and throat; the pain can last up to two hours and is usually worse after eating
- A sensation of food coming back into the mouth and leaving an acid or bitter taste
- Belching

When to Seek Help

- If your indigestion is accompanied by shortness of breath, sweating, or pain radiating to the jaw, neck, or arm ▶ *Seek emergency care immediately.*

- If your abdominal pain persists for several hours ▶ *Seek emergency care immediately.*

- If your chest pain is accompanied by sweating, light-headedness, and nausea ▶ *Seek emergency care immediately.*

- If your chest pain is sharp and severe or moves into your arms and shoulders ▶ *Seek emergency care immediately.*

- If taking an antacid does not relieve your burning chest pain within 15 minutes ▶ *Seek emergency care immediately.*

- If you have chronic indigestion or heartburn ▶ *Call your nurse information service or physician.*

Some people have functional indigestion. This type of indigestion happens when food is unable to move through the digestive tract.

Heartburn also has many causes. People with a digestive disorder, such as **gastritis**, often have heartburn. Other common causes of heartburn include being overweight, overeating, smoking, drinking too much alcohol or caffeine, and using nonsteroidal anti-inflammatory drugs such as aspirin and ibuprofen. Eating spicy, fatty, or acidic foods can also lead to heartburn.

Treatment

Most cases of indigestion and heartburn can be treated with lifestyle and dietary changes (see "At-Home Care" and "Prevention," below). Antacids can also provide temporary relief. They neutralize acid in the esophagus and stomach. If your indigestion or heartburn persists, you should see your physician for a complete diagnostic evaluation. Your physician may give you a prescription medication to help ease your discomfort.

At-Home Care

- Take an antacid.

- Avoid nonsteroidal anti-inflammatory drugs, such as aspirin and ibuprofen.

- Avoid heartburn "trigger" foods. These may include tomatoes, citrus fruits, coffee and tea, alcohol, peppermint-flavored food, chocolate, carbonated drinks, and fried and fatty foods.

> **CAUTION**
>
> If you have heart or kidney disease or **high blood pressure**, talk to your physician before taking an antacid. Also, antacids should not be taken for long periods of time. If you need antacids for more than two weeks, contact your physician.

- Sleep with your head raised six inches. You can raise the head of your bed by putting blocks or books under the feet of the headboard.

- Avoid lying down two to three hours after eating. If you must lie down, do so on your left side. (Your stomach will then be lower than your esophagus.)

Prevention

- Follow the tips under "At-Home Care."
- Maintain a healthy weight.
- Stop smoking, and avoid smoky places.
- Get plenty of exercise.
- Eat small, frequent meals rather than three large ones.

WHAT CAUSES GAS?
(And What You Can Do About It)

Everyone has digestive gas—and lots of it. In fact, most of us produce about 1 to 3 pints of gas each day. Some of it is absorbed into our bodies. We get rid of the rest of it by burping or by "passing gas." Most adults pass gas an average of 14 times a day.

Gas comes from two sources: swallowed air and the normal breakdown of certain foods by bacteria in the large intestine. Unfortunately, many of the foods that can cause excess gas—beans, vegetables, fruits, whole grains, and dairy products—are also very healthful. So rather than cutting down on these foods, try the following self-help measures to reduce gas:

• Eat and drink slowly.

• Do not chew gum.

• Avoid carbonated drinks.

• If you're trying to increase the fiber in your diet, do so slowly to give your body a chance to adjust.

• If you wear dentures, have them checked by your dentist. Loose-fitting dentures can cause you to swallow more air.

• Walk after eating. Mild exercise improves digestion.

• Try over-the-counter medications for gas. These include antacids with simethicone, activated charcoal tablets, and digestive enzymes. Your pharmacist can help you choose the right medication for you.

Sometimes gas can be a symptom of a more serious health concern. If your gas pains are severe or do not improve with the above self-help measures, call your physician.

Phlebitis

PHLEBITIS is an inflammation of the vein. The inflammation is sometimes accompanied by a blood clot, or *thrombus*, in the vein. When a blood clot is present, the condition is called *thrombophlebitis*—or sometimes phlebitis, for short.

A blood clot may partially or completely block the flow of blood in a vein. Sometimes this can cause pain and swelling. Or it may cause no symptoms at all. Age increases your risk for getting phlebitis. That's because older people tend to have more circulatory problems and vascular diseases. Such conditions can lead to phlebitis.

The most common type of phlebitis is called *superficial phlebitis*. It affects the veins visible just beneath the skin's surface. It is usually not dangerous and often heals with simple at-home treatment.

Deep vein phlebitis is a less common but much more serious condition. As its name implies, it affects veins deeper under the skin. These veins tend to be larger than ones near the skin's surface. The blood clots that form in them are larger, too—and more likely to break free and travel to the lungs. Clots that reach the lungs can cause serious, even life-threatening, breathing problems.

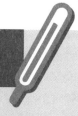

Symptoms

SUPERFICIAL PHLEBITIS

- A hard, cordlike vein on the surface of the leg that is very sensitive to pressure

- Swelling, throbbing, or burning sensation beneath the skin's surface

DEEP VEIN PHLEBITIS

- Aching pain and swelling throughout an entire arm or leg

- Bluish color in toes

Important: Many people with deep phlebitis have no symptoms at all.

When to Seek Help

- If you have symptoms of deep vein phlebitis (opposite)

  ▶ *Seek emergency care immediately.*

- If you have symptoms of superficial phlebitis (opposite)

  ▶ *Call your nurse information service or physician.*

Causes

Anyone who sits for long periods of time or needs prolonged bed rest, such as following surgery, is at increased risk for developing phlebitis. So are people who smoke, are overweight, or have **varicose veins**. A leg injury (from a blow or a fall) or a vein injury (from repeated intravenous injections) can also lead to phlebitis. In addition, women who take hormone replacement therapy for **menopause** may be at greater risk for developing both superficial and deep vein phlebitis.

Treatment

If you think you have any kind of phlebitis, you should see your physician for a diagnostic evaluation. Your physician may order X-rays, an ultrasound (a test that uses sound waves to locate clots), and other diagnostic tests to determine if deep veins are involved.

Treatment for superficial phlebitis usually involves resting the leg. To reduce pain and swelling, your physician may also suggest that you take a nonsteroidal anti-inflammatory medication, such as aspirin or ibuprofen.

If you are diagnosed with deep vein phlebitis, you may need to be hospitalized for several days. You will be treated with blood-thinning medications to prevent lung clots.

At-Home Care

(For Superficial Phlebitis)

- Rest the affected limb. Keep it raised above the level of your heart until the pain and swelling subside.

- Apply moist heat to the affected area.

- Take a nonsteroidal anti-inflammatory drug, such as aspirin or ibuprofen.

CAUTION

If you have phlebitis, do not massage the affected area. Rubbing the vein may dislodge a blood clot, which could eventually travel to your lungs.

- Try wearing elastic support stockings. They can improve blood flow and relieve pain and swelling.

Prevention

- Stop smoking.

- Exercise regularly.

- When taking a long auto or plane trip, be sure to get out of your seat and exercise your legs at least every two hours.

- Maintain a healthy weight.

- Never sit with your legs crossed.

- Avoid wearing knee-high stockings, tight pantyhose, and garters.

- If you are confined to bed, try this exercise: Put a pillow at the end of your bed against the footrest. Push your foot against it as if you were pushing against a gas pedal. Then release. Alternate from one foot to the other.

Pneumonia

PNEUMONIA happens when the lungs become infected or inflamed. Pus or other liquid fills the lungs, clogging the air sacs. This makes it difficult for oxygen to reach your blood. Without that oxygen, the cells in your body will not work properly. This can quickly become a life-threatening situation. The infection that caused the pneumonia may also spread through the body—sometimes with deadly results.

Until the mid-1930s, when antibiotics came into widespread use, pneumonia was the leading cause of death in the United States. Today it ranks sixth. For older people, however, pneumonia remains a serious health problem. People over age 65 are two to three times more likely to develop pneumonia than younger adults. They are also more likely to die from it.

Several factors explain this increased susceptibility. Older people often have weakened immune systems. They are also more likely to have a health problem, such as chronic lung disease or **diabetes**, that makes them more prone to pneumonia. And older people spend more time in hospitals. Strains of pneumonia picked up in hospitals tend to be more severe.

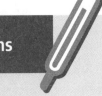

Symptoms

- Fever, cough, **headaches**, muscle pain, and weakness

- Shortness of breath

- Chest pain that worsens when breathing deeply

- A cough that produces rust-colored or greenish mucus

- Abdominal pain, nausea, vomiting

- Shaking chills and sweating

- Bluish lips and nails

- Extreme fatigue

- Confusion

- Delirium

When to Seek Help

- If you develop bluish lips and nails with any other symptoms of pneumonia (p. 167)

  ▶ *Seek emergency care immediately.*

- If you or a family member or loved one with symptoms of a cold or flu becomes suddenly confused or delirious

  ▶ *Seek emergency care immediately.*

- If your symptoms indicate you have pneumonia (p. 167)

  ▶ *Call your nurse information service or physician.*

Causes

The most common causes of pneumonia are as follows:

- Viruses. Many viruses can invade the lungs and cause pneumonia. Viral pneumonias are usually mild and last a short time. However, those caused by the flu virus can be severe and, in some cases, deadly. People with a preexisting heart or lung disease are particularly at risk.

- Bacteria. Several different kinds of bacteria can infect the lungs and cause pneumonia. *Streptococcus pneumoniae*, sometimes called pneumococcus, is the most common cause of bacterial pneumonia. It can trigger a very serious type of pneumonia, especially among older people and those with chronic illnesses.

- Fungi. Some types of fungi can be inhaled into the lungs and cause pneumonia. One organism believed to be a fungus, *Pneumocystis carinii*, is a common cause of pneumonia in people with **AIDS**.

Treatment

Chances for recovery from pneumonia are greatest when the illness is caught early. So if you suspect you have pneumonia, see your physician for a diagnostic evaluation as soon as possible.

The treatment you receive will depend on what kind of pneumonia you have and how severe it is. It will also depend on whether you have any preexisting health conditions. Viral pneumonia is usually treated with bed rest, fluids, and medications for pain and fever. If you have bacterial pneumonia, your physician will probably prescribe an antibiotic. If your illness is caused by a fungus, you may be given an antifungal medication.

Most people can recover from pneumonia at home. But if your lungs are severely congested, you may need to be hospitalized.

At-Home Care

- Get plenty of rest and sleep.

- Drink lots of fluids.

- Avoid cough suppressants during the day if you are coughing up mucus. The coughing will help you recover.

- Apply heat to your chest to reduce pain. Use a heating pad or a hot-water bottle wrapped in a towel. Apply the heat in 10-minute intervals. Repeat several times a day.

Prevention

- Get a flu shot each year. Also, if you are aged 65 or older, be sure you have been immunized against pneumococcal pneumonia. (For more information about immunizations, see p. 42.)

- Stop smoking, and avoid smoky areas. Smoking weakens your ability to fight the viruses and bacteria that cause pneumonia.

- Watch your alcohol consumption. Heavy drinking of alcohol can also weaken your immune system.

- Exercise daily. Exercise helps keep the immune system strong.

- Avoid close, prolonged exposure to people who have **colds**.

Sexually Transmitted Diseases

IF you are sexually active, you are at risk for developing a sexually transmitted disease (STD). Age does not protect you. Nor does being in a mutually faithful relationship—not if your partner has been previously infected. Many people who are infected don't know it, and some people are not honest about their sexual history.

Once known as venereal diseases, STDs are contracted by means of vaginal, anal, or oral sex. Medical experts have identified more than 20 types of STDs. The most common ones are *chlamydia, gonorrhea, syphilis, genital herpes*, and *genital warts*. **HIV**, the virus that causes **AIDS**, is also an STD.

Most bacterial STDs (see below) can be cured or managed if diagnosed and treated early. Unfortunately, many people do not develop noticeable symptoms until some permanent damage has occurred. STDs can adversely affect more than your reproductive system. They can also damage your heart, eyes, brain, and other organs. Having an STD also weakens your immune system. This leaves you more vulnerable to other infections.

Causes

Some STDs are caused by bacteria. These include chlamydia, gonorrhea, and syphilis. Other STDs—such as genital herpes, genital

Symptoms

- Abnormal or smelly discharge from the vagina, penis, or rectum

- Genital and/or anal itching

- Blisters, boils, sores, lumps, warts, or a rash in the genital area

- Burning during urination

- Vaginal bleeding

- Pain or swelling in the groin or lower abdomen

- Testicular swelling

- Pain during intercourse

- Fatigue and flulike symptoms

warts, and **HIV**—are caused by viruses. People who have more than one sex partner, who do not use a latex condom when having sex, or who have sex with IV drug users are at high risk for developing an STD.

Treatment

If you are in a high-risk category, you should be tested for STDs during an annual health examination with your physician. Ask for the tests. Some physicians do not automatically test older people for STDs.

When to Seek Help

• If you are experiencing any of the symptoms of sexually transmitted diseases (opposite)

▼

Call your nurse information service or physician.

If you have a bacterial STD, you will be treated with antibiotics. Bacterial STDs can usually be cured if treatment is started early enough. There are no cures for viral STDs. But their symptoms can be managed with medication.

If you are diagnosed with an STD, your sexual partners will need to be treated, too.

Prevention

• Have sex with only a mutually faithful partner who has tested negative for STDs twice over a six-month interval.

• Practice "safer sex": If you have sex with more than one partner, use latex condoms and a water-based lubricant. Women whose male partners don't use condoms can help protect themselves with a female condom. Talk to your physician about safer sex. Don't be embarrassed. A healthy sex life is an important part of total health.

• Select your sexual partners carefully. Find out about the person's health and sexual history before you have sex, but understand that you must still practice safer sex each and every time. No method of protection against STDs is 100 percent effective.

- Always avoid sex with someone who has a genital sore, rash, or other STD symptom.

- If you think you have been exposed to an STD, see your physician for testing and treatment. Make sure your partner is tested and treated, too.

How Will Having an STD Change My Life?

Having an STD will affect your sexual behavior. You will have to refrain from sex with a partner until your physician says it's safe. If you have an STD that cannot be cured, you will have to take preventive measures each time you have sex in the future to minimize the risk of spreading the disease to a partner. (See "Prevention," p. 171.) However, be aware that no method offers 100 percent protection.

Discovering you have contracted a sexually transmitted disease can be an emotional experience. You may feel embarrassment, shock, anger, even fear. Usually those intense feelings go away with time and as you gain more knowledge about how to treat and manage your disease. If the feelings persist, however, you may benefit from talking with a psychologist or other qualified counselor about your concerns.

Living with **HIV** or **AIDS** can be particularly devastating, for both you and your loved ones. Fortunately, many organizations offer support to people with this disease. Ask your physician for referrals, or contact the organizations listed in the "Resources" section of this book.

Sexual Problems

SEXUAL enjoyment and satisfaction need not decline with age. For many people, sexual activity, which includes touching and caressing, continues through their 70s, 80s, and beyond. In fact, most older people are able to have an active, satisfying sex life.

Sometimes, however, illness, disability, medications, or **depression** and other emotional disorders can lead to sexual problems. These problems rarely threaten a person's health, but they can have a devastating psychological impact. They can also affect your relationship with your spouse or partner.

Sexual problems can take many forms. The most common problems in older men are difficulty achieving or maintaining an erection (*impotence*) and early or delayed ejaculation. The most common sexual problems experienced by older women are pain during intercourse (*dyspareunia*) and diminished arousal.

Causes

As your body ages, it goes through some normal changes that can influence your sexual response. After **menopause**, a woman's vagina takes longer to lubricate during arousal. The opening may also narrow.

Symptoms

MEN

- Premature ejaculation

- Delayed ejaculation

- Inability to have an erection (impotence)

- Pain during intercourse

- Lack or loss of sexual desire

- Persistent painful erection (*priapism*)

WOMEN

- Lack or loss of sexual desire

- Difficulty achieving orgasm

- Pain or discomfort during intercourse

When to Seek Help

- If you have sexual problems that are causing you concern

  ▶ *Call your nurse information service or physician.*

- If you are experiencing pain during intercourse

  ▶ *Call your nurse information service or physician.*

These factors can lead to difficult or painful intercourse. Also, the amount of blood that flows to a woman's genitals may diminish as she ages. This means it may take longer for the tissues to become *engorged*, or swollen with blood, during arousal. Orgasms may therefore take longer to develop or be less intense.

The flow of blood in men also lessens with age. This can result in slower, smaller, and softer erections. The feeling that an ejaculation is about to happen may last for a shorter time. Erections may also disappear more rapidly after orgasm. And it may take longer before another erection is possible.

Several illnesses and disabilities can also lead to sexual problems. About 70 percent of cases of male impotence, for example, are caused by **diabetes**, kidney disease, chronic **alcoholism**, multiple sclerosis, atherosclerosis, and vascular disease. Surgery—for prostate disease, for example—can also injure nerves and arteries in a way that can cause sexual problems. But even the most serious medical condition need not stop you from having a satisfying sex life. (See "Effects of Illness or Disability," opposite.)

In addition, certain medications, including drugs for **high blood pressure**, antihistamines, antidepressants, tranquilizers, appetite suppressants, and cimetidine (a drug for **stomach ulcers**), have been linked to sexual problems. And smoking, which affects the flow of blood in the body, also contributes to sexual dysfunction.

Some sexual problems have emotional roots. Significant changes—such as retirement, moving into a new living situation, dating, children leaving home, death of parents—can lead to **anxiety**, stress, or sadness. All these emotions can affect sexual performance and enjoyment. Older men sometimes worry so much about impotence that the stress from their concern causes it to happen. Both men and women may become more anxious about their appearance as they age. They may believe they are no longer "attractive"—a feeling that may interfere with their ability to enjoy sex.

Treatment

If you are having concerns about your sexual life, discuss them with your physician. Don't feel embarrassed; a healthy sex life is an important part of total health. Your physician will ask you questions, review your medical history, and try to assess your symptoms. Sexual problems can almost always be treated. If your physician tells you to "live with it" or that "it's to be expected," find a new physician. The problem may have a physical source that your physician can diagnose and treat. Or the problem may be resolved by switching to a different medication. Sexual aids, such as lubricants for a dry vagina (available over the counter at drugstores), can also help. So can learning new sexual techniques. Many couples find that the increased length of time for arousal and climax offers them more sensual opportunities.

Many treatment options exist for chronic male impotence. These treatments include psychotherapy, drug therapy, injections, vacuum devices that cause erections by creating a partial vacuum around the penis, and surgery.

If you feel your sexual problems have a psychological or emotional source, talking to a psychologist or trained counselor may help. Some therapists specialize in treating sexual problems. Ask your physician for a referral.

Effects of Illness or Disability

- **Diabetes**. Most people with **diabetes** do not have sexual problems. The disease can cause impotence in men, however. And women with **diabetes** may be more likely to have sexual problems than women without the disease. Changes in blood vessels and nerve damage caused by **diabetes** are believed to be the cause. Medical treatment may help in some cases.

- **Coronary heart disease**. Heart disease can affect small blood vessels and restrict blood flow to your genitals. This can interfere with a man's erection and a woman's arousal. Treating the illness, however, can often resolve the problem. Many people with **coronary heart disease**, especially if they have had a heart attack, worry that having sex will cause another attack. The risk is very low. Heart attack survivors usually can resume sexual activity as soon as they feel ready to do so. Talk to your physician first.

- **Stroke**. Most people who have had a **stroke** do not lose any of their physical ability to function sexually. It is also unlikely that sexual exertion will cause another **stroke**. If a **stroke** has caused weakness or paralysis, using different positions or medical devices can help. Talk to your physician.

- **Arthritis**. Some people with **arthritis** find their sexual activity limited by joint pain. Medications and surgery may relieve this pain. In some cases, however, the medications may actually decrease sexual desire. Resting or taking a warm shower or bath before sex can be helpful. Also, try using different positions, and time sexual encounters for those periods of the day when pain is at its lowest.

- Prostatectomy (surgical removal of all or part of a man's prostate). Today this procedure rarely causes impotence. New surgical techniques can often remove the prostate without cutting nerves that control penile erection. If impotence does occur, it can often be overcome with devices that aid erection or with a penile implant. New drugs can also help. Discuss all your options with your physician before the surgery.

- Hysterectomy (surgical removal of a woman's uterus). Usually, a hysterectomy does not hinder sexual functioning, although some women report that intercourse feels different afterward. Nor does this operation generally decrease a woman's sexual desire. If you are having sexual problems after a hysterectomy, you may benefit from talking to a trained therapist or counselor. Ask your physician for a referral.

- Mastectomy (surgical removal of all or part of a woman's breast). Having a mastectomy should not affect your sexual response. Many women feel less attractive or confident about their sexuality after this surgery, however. This can lead to a loss of sexual desire. Talk about this with your partner. Bring your concerns out into the open. Most women are surprised to find that their partners don't find them any less attractive. You may find it useful to talk to a trained therapist or counselor about your concerns. Talking with other women who have had a mastectomy may also be useful. Contact your local chapter of the American Cancer Society and ask for information about their Reach for Recovery program.

Prevention

- Don't let sexual difficulties fester because you're embarrassed or believe they're an inevitable sign of aging. Talk to your partner and your physician at the first sign of difficulty.

- Exercise regularly. It can help reduce your risk for **coronary heart disease** and **diabetes**, two illnesses that can lead to sexual problems. People who stay in shape also tend to have more energy, stamina, and flexibility.

- Eat a low-fat, high-fiber diet. Make sure it includes lots of vegetables, fruits, and whole grains.

- Maintain a healthful weight.

- Don't smoke, and avoid excessive amounts of alcohol.

- Reduce stress. Learn relaxation techniques. Massage can also be very helpful—especially if performed by your partner.

- Schedule regular health checkups with your physician.

Skin Concerns

Our skin changes as we age. It becomes less flexible, thinner, drier, and more wrinkled. Spots and growths may appear. Older skin also takes longer to heal.

Many of these changes are natural and unavoidable. Some, however, can cause pain or discomfort. A few, such as skin cancers, pose a serious health problem and require immediate medical attention.

Symptoms

AGE SPOTS

- Flat, brown spots on the face, back, hands, or feet

DRY SKIN

- Flaky and itchy skin

PURPURAS (BRUISES)

- Reddish-brown or purplish marks anywhere on the body

SEBORRHEIC KERATOSES

- Slightly raised, light brown spots that gradually darken, thicken, and develop a rough, wartlike surface

SHINGLES

- Pain, itching, or tenderness in an area of skin, usually on only one side of the face or body
- One to three days later: a painful, red, blistering rash on same area of skin

SKIN CANCER

- A mole or other darkly pigmented area that changes its size, color, shape, or texture
- A scaly red spot
- Any new skin growth
- Bleeding in a mole or other growth

Age Spots

The medical name for these small, flat, brown spots is *lentigines*. Many people call them "liver spots," although they have nothing to do with the liver. They usually occur on the face, back, hands, and feet. Almost everyone over the age of 55 has them.

Causes and Treatment

Age spots are caused by the sun. They develop over many years and are a sign of sun damage. Age spots are harmless and do not need to be treated. If you dislike their appearance, however, you can have them lightened or removed. Talk to your physician or a *dermatologist* (a physician who specializes in the treatment of diseases and problems of the skin). Treatments for age spots include prescription "fade" medications that are applied to the skin, acid peels, and laser therapies.

Dry Skin

Dry skin is a common problem for older adults, especially those who live in cold, dry, windy climates. In fact, about 85 percent of older people develop "winter itch," a condition caused by dry, overheated indoor air. Because dry skin can be easily irritated, it often itches. Severe itching can make you anxious and interfere with your sleep. Repeated scratching of the skin can also lead to an infection.

Causes

Our skin becomes drier as we age because it loses some of its sweat and oil glands. Other factors can contribute to the problem. These include overusing soaps, antiperspirants, and perfumes, or bathing in overheated water.

Treatment

Using a moisturizer after bathing, while the skin is still damp, can help relieve dry skin. Moisturizers that contain petrolatum or lanolin are particularly effective in sealing in moisture. Bathing less often and using milder soaps or a soap substitute can also help. When you do bathe or shower, use warm rather than hot water; warm water is less irritating to the skin.

If you live in a dry climate, use an indoor humidifier to keep the air inside your home moist. Drinking plenty of water will also help add moisture to your skin.

If dry skin continues to be a problem for you, see your physician. Severely flaky, itchy, and cracked skin may be a sign of an underlying health problem.

When to Seek Help

• If you have shingles (p. 178) and the rash spreads to your face	▶ *Call your nurse information service or physician immediately.*
• If you have shingles (p. 178) other than on your face	▶ *Call your nurse information service or physician.*
• If a mole changes size, color, shape, or texture	▶ *Call your nurse information service or physician.*
• If you have an open sore on your skin that does not heal	▶ *Call your nurse information service or physician.*
• If you have severely flaky, itchy, and cracked skin	▶ *Call your nurse information service or physician.*
• If you develop red, painful, fluid-filled blisters	▶ *Call your nurse information service or physician.*
• If you bruise often and easily, for no apparent reason	▶ *Call your nurse information service or physician.*
• If a bruise does not fade or go away within 14 days	▶ *Call your nurse information service or physician.*
• If your skin problem does not respond to treatment	▶ *Call your nurse information service or physician.*

Purpuras (Bruises)

Many older people develop spontaneous reddish-brown or purplish bruises—called *purpuras*—particularly on their arms and legs. These spots may grow as large as two inches across.

Causes

Purpuras are caused by bleeding under the skin. When skin ages it becomes thinner, losing some of its fat and connective tissue. As a result, blood vessels are less "cushioned," making them more prone to injury.

Medications that interfere with blood clotting and several internal diseases can also cause bruises to form. A bruise near a bone may indicate a fracture. You should have any unexplainable bruises checked out by your physician.

Treatment

Most purpuras heal on their own, but deep or large ones may require medical care. Treatment will depend on the underlying cause of the bruising.

Seborrheic Keratoses

Sometimes called "the barnacles of aging," seborrheic keratoses are harmless skin growths that are common among older people. They begin as slightly raised, light brown spots. Over time they darken, thicken, and develop a rough, wartlike surface. They can also grow as large as a silver dollar. These changes are harmless.

AT-HOME CARE FOR DRY SKIN

- Use a humidifier to keep indoor air from getting too dry.
- Use an unscented moisturizer after bathing or showering.
- Take fewer, cooler baths and showers.
- Drink plenty of water.

Causes

The cause of seborrheic keratoses is unknown. The tendency to develop these growths appears to be inherited; light-skinned people are particularly prone to getting them.

Treatment

Seborrheic keratoses do not need to be treated. You may choose to have them removed, however, if you find the growths unattractive or if they cause you discomfort. Removal can be done surgically or by *cryotherapy* (freezing them with liquid nitrogen). Your physician will suggest the method that is best for you.

Shingles

Shingles is a painful, blistery skin rash that usually strikes only one side of the face or body. It begins with a burning or itching sensation, which is followed one to three days later by the rash. After one to two weeks the blisters dry and form scabs, although the pain may continue.

You can develop shingles at any age, but it is most common in people over age 50. Half of people over age 85 have had it.

Shingles can involve nerves to the eye and, in rare cases, can lead to blindness. Blisters on the nose are an early sign that the eyes may be affected. If you experience eye pain with your rash or if the rash spreads to your face, contact your physician immediately.

Causes

To get shingles you must first have had chicken pox earlier in your life. That's because shingles is caused by the same virus that causes chicken pox. Here's what happens: The virus does not go away when the chicken pox sores heal. Instead it lies dormant in nerve cells near the spine. Then years—even decades—later, the virus becomes reactivated.

Scientists don't know why the virus becomes reactivated in some people and not in others. But people whose immune systems are weakened by a chronic illness, such as **AIDS** or **cancer**, are more likely to get shingles. Some medications also raise the risk for developing this skin rash.

Treatment

Shingles is usually treated with antiviral drugs. Your physician may also prescribe pain medication and corticosteroids to reduce inflammation. If the rash becomes infected with bacteria, you may also be given antibiotics.

Skin Cancer

Skin cancer is the most common form of **cancer** in the United States. More than 700,000 Americans are diagnosed with skin cancer annually. About 9,000 people die from the disease. The National Institutes of Health estimates that 40 to 50 percent of Americans who live to age 65 will have skin cancer at least once.

Fortunately, skin cancer is curable if it is detected and treated at an early stage. That's why it's so important to examine yourself every month for signs of skin cancer—and to see your physician promptly if you find something suspicious.

There are three common types of skin cancers:

- Basal cell carcinomas are the most common. They often appear as small, smooth, shiny, pale, or waxy lumps. Others look like firm red lumps or flat red spots. They grow slowly, seldom spread beyond the skin, and thus are rarely life-threatening.

- Squamous cell carcinomas are less common. They look like basal cell carcinomas and are also slow growing. But these cancers can spread—and be fatal—if not treated in their earliest stages.

- Melanomas are the most dangerous of all skin cancers. They appear as changes in existing moles or in other pigmented areas of the skin. They also sometimes show up as scaly red spots. Melanomas can quickly spread beyond the skin to other organs. Once they do this, they are very difficult to treat. Fortunately, most cases of melanoma can be cured if treatment is begun early.

Causes

The main cause of skin cancer is excessive exposure to the sun's ultraviolet (UV) radiation. Anyone can get skin cancer, but some people are at greater risk. These include people with red or blond hair, blue or light-colored eyes, and fair skin that freckles or burns rather than tans. You are also at increased risk if you live in a sunny climate, work outdoors, or have a personal or family history of skin cancer. In addition, having a large number of moles or atypical moles—ones that are unusually large or irregular in shape or color—puts you at greater risk.

Diagnosis and Treatment

If you notice any unusual changes in your skin, you should see your physician. To determine whether a skin growth is cancer, it must be *biopsied*, or surgically removed and studied under a microscope. If the growth is cancerous, your physician may order other tests to determine if the cancer has spread.

Treatment for skin cancer depends on the type and stage of the disease. If the tumor has not spread, all that may be required is simple removal of the cancerous tissue. But if the tumor has spread beyond the skin, other treatments, such as radiation or drug therapy (chemotherapy), may be needed.

Skin Cancer Prevention

- Check your skin—especially moles—regularly for changes. Think "ABC": Look for changes in the **A**symmetry, **B**order, and **C**olor of the mole.

- Promptly report any suspicious changes or new growths on your skin to your physician.

- Avoid unnecessary sun exposure—especially between 10 A.M. and 3 P.M., when UV rays are strongest.

- When outdoors, wear protective clothing, such as long-sleeved shirts, hats, and sunglasses that block UV rays.

- Use a sunscreen with a sun protection factor (SPF) of 15 or higher when outdoors.

- Do not use artificial tanning devices, such as sun lamps or tanning booths. They can be more dangerous than the sun.

Sleep Problems

SLEEP problems are very common, particularly among older people. As we age, we tend to sleep more lightly and for shorter periods of time. But we still need to get a good night's sleep. Not getting enough sleep can leave us feeling tired and irritable during the day. Our judgment and reaction time also lessen, making us more prone to accidents.

Sleep problems often begin in middle age. Experts estimate that about half of all people over age 65 have frequent sleeping problems. In some cases those problems may be a normal part of aging. Often, however, sleep problems are the result of

Symptoms

INSOMNIA

- Difficulty falling asleep
- Difficulty staying asleep
- Early waking
- Daytime sleepiness

SLEEP APNEA

- Loud snoring with or without long pauses
- Periodic episodes of struggling for air while sleeping
- Excessive daytime sleepiness

RESTLESS LEGS SYNDROME

- Unpleasant crawling, tingling, or sometimes painful feelings in the legs, usually just before or during sleep
- Uncontrollable twitching of the legs (and sometimes of the arms)
- A strong, constant urge to move the feet and legs

When to Seek Help

- If you have had trouble sleeping for more than two weeks
  ▶ *Call your nurse information service or physician.*

- If you have symptoms of sleep apnea (p. 185)
  ▶ *Call your nurse information service or physician.*

- If you feel sleepy all the time
  ▶ *Call your nurse information service or physician.*

other illnesses or medications used to treat those illnesses. Mcst sleep disorders can be treated. So talk to your doctor if you are having trouble sleeping.

More than 70 sleep disorders have been identified. The most common ones among older adults are *insomnia, sleep apnea,* and *restless legs syndrome.*

Insomnia

Insomnia—difficulty falling or staying asleep—is the most common sleep complaint. It affects about 60 million Americans each year.

Causes

Short-term insomnia is usually caused by stress or a change in habits or schedule. But if the insomnia persists for more than a few weeks, it may be a sign of a medical problem. Some common medical causes of insomnia include **depression, arthritis, heartburn, menopause, diabetes, thyroid problems, chronic obstructive pulmonary disease, Parkinson's disease**, and **Alzheimer's disease**. Alcohol and drug abuse can also disrupt sleep.

Many medications can adversely affect sleep. Some drugs commonly linked to insomnia include antidepressants, steroids, beta-blockers, and decongestants. If you develop sleep problems after starting a new medication, talk to your physician.

Treatment

You may be able to overcome mild insomnia by following good sleep habits. (See "Tips for Getting a Good Night's Sleep," p. 188.) For more serious sleep disorders, see your physician for a thorough medical examination. If your insomnia is due to an underlying medical condition, treating that condition may help. Your physician may also refer you to a sleep disorder center or clinic for further testing and treatment.

Sleep Apnea

Sleep apnea is a disorder in which breathing becomes interrupted during sleep. People with this disorder may stop breathing dozens of times a night and not know it. They are often (but not always) loud snorers and feel extremely sleepy during the day.

Most of the estimated 18 million Americans with sleep apnea are unaware they have the problem. Usually it's a spouse or other loved one who first notices the person struggling for air during sleep—or struggling to stay awake during the day. Sleep apnea is sometimes associated with serious health problems, including **coronary heart disease**. If you have symptoms of the disorder, see your physician right away.

Causes

Sleep apnea occurs when the muscles in the throat relax, briefly blocking the airways in the throat. People who are overweight or who have a physical abnormality in the nose, throat, or other part of the upper airway are more likely to develop the disorder. Sleep apnea is most common among men. It also tends to run in families.

Diagnosis and Treatment

For a proper diagnosis, you will need to spend a night in a sleep clinic. You will be given a test called a *polysomnography*, which records brain waves, heartbeat, and breathing during an entire night. Mild sleep apnea is often treated with weight loss and with techniques that prevent the person from sleeping on his or her back. Devices worn during sleep to keep the airway open are also available. More severe cases require surgery to correct the obstruction. People with sleep apnea should never take sleeping pills; such medication may keep them from waking up enough to breathe.

TIPS FOR GETTING A GOOD NIGHT'S SLEEP

- Get up about the same time every day.
- Go to bed only when you are sleepy.
- Establish relaxing presleep rituals, such as a warm bath, a light bedtime snack, or 10 minutes of reading.
- Exercise regularly. If you exercise vigorously, do this at least six hours before bedtime. Mild exercise—such as simple stretching or walking—should not be done within four hours of bedtime.
- Maintain a regular schedule. Regular times for eating meals, taking medications, doing chores, and performing other activities help keep your "inner clock" running smoothly.

- Don't eat or drink anything containing caffeine within six hours of bedtime. Don't drink alcohol within several hours of bedtime or when you are sleepy. Tiredness can intensify the effects of alcohol.
- Avoid smoking close to bedtime.
- If you take naps, try to do so at the same time every day. For most people, a midafternoon nap is most helpful.
- Avoid sleeping pills, or use them conservatively. Most physicians avoid prescribing sleeping pills for a period of longer than three weeks. Never drink alcohol while taking sleeping pills.

Source: American Academy of Sleep Medicine

Restless Legs Syndrome

People with this disorder experience unpleasant creepy, crawly, or tingling sensations deep in their legs or feet. The feelings are often especially strong at night, right before or during sleep. Many people also experience involuntary jerking or bending leg movements during sleep. These twitches may occur every 10 to 60 seconds.

Restless legs syndrome can strike at any age, but it is most common in older adults. People with the disorder have great difficulty falling and staying asleep—and experience excessive sleepiness during the day.

Causes

The cause of restless legs syndrome is unknown. It appears, however, to run in families. People who have anemia, or low levels of iron in their blood, have an increased risk for developing the syndrome. So do people with **diabetes**, rheumatoid **arthritis**, and kidney disease.

Treatment

Mild cases of restless legs syndrome can often be helped with simple at-home treatments, such as taking warm baths, massaging the legs, exercising, and eliminating caffeine from the diet. Medications can help more severe cases. Some people have also found a treatment called *transcutaneous electric nerve stimulation* helpful. This technique involves applying electrical stimulation to the legs for 15 to 30 minutes, usually before bedtime.

How Will Having a Sleep Disorder Change My Life?

Not getting enough sleep can profoundly affect how well—or how poorly—you function during your waking hours. Sleepless nights can lead to **depression, high blood pressure**, irritability, **sexual problems**, an increased risk of automobile and other accidents, and learning and memory difficulties. It can also lead to excessive daytime sleepiness and fatigue, which can interfere with the quality of your life and your relationships with others.

Most people with sleep disorders are unaware that they have a problem. Or they may not seek help out of a mistaken belief that "nothing can be done." But sleeping poorly is not an inevitable part of aging. Help is available. If you are having trouble sleeping or feel excessively sleepy during the day, talk to your physician. Or contact a sleep center or clinic in your area.

Stomach Ulcers and Gastritis

A stomach ulcer (also called a *peptic ulcer*) is an open, craterlike sore in the lining of the gastrointestinal tract. The problem starts when the normally protective lining becomes damaged. This allows stomach acids and enzymes to eat away at it, creating a sore. Ulcers that develop in the stomach are *gastric ulcers*; those that develop in the upper part of the small intestine (the duodenum) are *duodenal ulcers*. Only rarely do ulcers develop in the esophagus (the tube that leads from the throat to the stomach).

Many people are unaware they have ulcers because they have no symptoms. If they do experience a symptom, it is often a gnawing pain in the upper abdomen that happens soon after eating. The pain may be relieved by eating. If the pain becomes severe, it may be a sign of a perforated ulcer (an ulcer that has completely penetrated the lining of the stomach or duodenum). A perforated ulcer can be life-threatening and may require emergency surgery. If you experience sharp abdominal pain, seek emergency care immediately.

Gastritis is an inflammation of the stomach lining. Symptoms may include upper abdominal pain, nausea, vomiting, diarrhea, fatigue, and loss of appetite. Attacks of gastritis can be either acute, lasting

Symptoms

- Dull, aching pain in the upper abdomen about an hour after eating; the pain is often temporarily relieved by eating or drinking something
- **Indigestion**
- **Heartburn**
- Nausea or vomiting
- Fatigue
- Dark or bloody stools
- Weight loss, in some people

Important: Many people with stomach ulcers have no symptoms at all.

190

When to Seek Help

• If you vomit blood or anything that looks like coffee grounds	▶ *Seek emergency care immediately.*
• If you pass bloody or black, tarry stools	▶ *Seek emergency care immediately.*
• If you experience signs of shock— for example, if you feel faint, chilly, or sweaty	▶ *Seek emergency care immediately.*
• If you have intense abdominal pain	▶ *Seek emergency care immediately.*
• If you have symptoms of a stomach ulcer or gastritis (opposite) that last more than several days	▶ *Call your nurse information service or physician.*

only one or two days, or chronic, continuing for many weeks or months. People with chronic gastritis often have no abdominal pain but may experience a loss of appetite or nausea.

Causes

The prime cause of stomach ulcers and gastritis is an infection by a common bacterium, *Helicobacter pylori*. Most people over age 60 have the bacterium in their digestive tract; but for unknown reasons it does not cause infections in everyone. Long-term use of steroid medications, aspirin, and nonsteroidal anti-inflammatory drugs can also break down the stomach lining and increase the risk for getting ulcers or gastritis. Stress and spicy foods do *not* cause either condition, but they can worsen the symptoms. So can drinking alcohol and caffeine, or smoking.

The likelihood of developing stomach ulcers and gastritis increases with age. Scientists believe this may be because older people tend to take more aspirin and other medications that can irritate the stomach lining.

Treatment

Mild cases are usually treated with over-the-counter or prescription drugs, such as antacids, that reduce stomach acid or coat the stomach lining. If bacteria are the problem, you will be given antibiotics as well as acid relievers. In severe cases surgery may be needed to stop internal bleeding and repair any perforations in the stomach wall.

At-Home Care

- Avoid aspirin, ibuprofen, and other nonsteroidal anti-inflammatory drugs. If you need a pain reliever, use acetaminophen.

- Take antacids. *Caution:* Regular use of antacids can worsen kidney problems and interfere with some medications. Talk to your physician before using them.

- Drink plenty of water to prevent dehydration. But avoid milk, which can increase acid.

- Eat smaller meals. Avoid foods that cause symptoms.

- Do not smoke. Smoking slows the healing process. It also increases the likelihood of the ulcers returning.

- Avoid alcohol.

- Avoid caffeinated beverages if you are sensitive to them.

Prevention

- Follow the tips under "At-Home Care," above.

- Eat more high-fiber foods. Fiber helps produce a bodily secretion called *mucin*, which protects the duodenal lining. (For a list of high-fiber foods, see p. 5.)

Urinary Incontinence

INCONTINENCE is loss of bladder control or involuntary leakage of urine. It can happen to people of any age but is very common among older people. At least 1 in 10 people over the age of 65 have some type of urinary incontinence. Women are affected more often than men.

Incontinence can range from mild leaking of urine to severe and uncontrollable wetting. It can sometimes lead to **bladder and other urinary tract infections**. The leakage may also cause skin rashes. Despite its rather mild symptoms, urinary incontinence is considered a major health problem because it can lead to disability and dependence. This is particularly true for older people. In fact, urinary incontinence is a major reason older people are placed in nursing homes.

Fortunately, most cases of urinary incontinence are curable, or at least treatable. If you are having bladder control problems, see your physician. Even if your incontinence cannot be completely cured, you can learn to manage it in a way that will enable you to continue an active life.

(Incontinence of bowels is also a problem for some older people. If you are having a problem controlling your bowels, be sure to discuss it with your doctor.)

Symptoms

- Inability to hold back urine, resulting in dribbling or leaking
- An urgent need to urinate

Causes

Although urinary incontinence is common among older people, it is not an inevitable consequence of aging. Changes that occur with the natural aging process may, however, contribute to the problem.

When to Seek Help

- If you are having bladder control problems ▶ *Call your nurse information service or physician.*

- If you have any pain when you urinate ▶ *Call your nurse information service or physician.*

The many causes of incontinence include the following:

- Infection
- **Constipation**
- Weak or overactive bladder muscles
- Nerve damage
- Large fibroid or ovarian tumor (in women)
- Decline in estrogen that occurs after **menopause** (in women)
- Enlargement of the prostate gland (in men)
- Various illnesses, such as **diabetes, stroke, Parkinson's disease**, multiple sclerosis, and **Alzheimer's disease**
- Certain medications, such as sedatives, antihistamines, diuretics, and tranquilizers

Diagnosis and Treatment

If you are having bladder control problems, see your physician. He or she will give you a complete medical evaluation. The exam may include urine tests. Your physician may then refer you to a *urologist*. This physician specializes in the treatment of diseases involving the urinary tract.

The type of treatment your physician recommends will depend on what is causing your bladder problems. Often, simple lifestyle changes—such as eating more high-fiber foods to avoid **constipation** or reducing the amount of caffeine and alcohol you drink—can eliminate the problem. Your physician may also want to change the dosage of some of your medications or give you an antibiotic if you have an infection.

For persistent cases of incontinence, your physician will probably recommend that you try behavioral treatments. Many people find bladder training helpful. It involves urinating at scheduled intervals—usually every 30 or 60 minutes. The intervals are then gradually increased to several hours. *Biofeedback*—a technique that uses sophisticated equipment to teach people how to control various physiological functions—can also help you regain control of your bladder.

Several devices are used to treat incontinence in women. One of the newest of these devices is the *disposable urethral plug*, which fits inside the urethra to stop leakage. Various medications, designed to help strengthen the muscles involved in urination, are also prescribed for incontinence.

If none of these treatments works, your physician may recommend surgery. Surgery is particularly successful if the incontinence is caused by a structural problem, such as an abnormally positioned bladder or blockage due to an enlarged prostate.

What is…?

…stress incontinence? This is the most common type of incontinence, particularly among women. It happens when a sneeze, cough, laugh, or any other activity puts pressure on the bladder, causing urine to leak.

…urge incontinence? With this type of incontinence, the person is unable to control the urge to urinate.

…mixed incontinence? This is a combination of both stress and urge incontinence.

…overflow incontinence? With this type of incontinence, the person is unable to completely empty the bladder. As a result, the bladder is always a little bit full. Urine dribbles out. Overflow incontinence is more common in men than in women.

…unconscious or reflex incontinence? People with this type of incontinence have no sensory awareness, or warning, that they are about to lose urine.

…functional incontinence? This happens in people who have normal bladder control but can't get to the toilet in time because of **arthritis** or some other physical problem.

195

At-Home Care

- Keep a written record of when you lose control of your bladder. Make note of what you were doing at the time. Take this information with you when you visit your physician. It will help you and your physician develop an effective treatment plan.

- Eliminate coffee, tea, or other caffeinated drinks from your diet. They can irritate the bladder.

- Don't smoke. Nicotine can irritate the bladder.

- Try bladder training. Slowly increase the intervals between trips to the bathroom.

- For women who have stress incontinence: Cross your legs when sneezing or coughing. This simple practice may prevent leakage.

- Wear special underwear or pads that absorb moisture. Change these supplies often to prevent skin rashes.

Prevention

- Keep your weight down. Excess pounds can put pressure on your bladder muscles.

- For women: Practice Kegel exercises daily to strengthen the muscles that control urine flow. You can identify the muscles you need to exercise while you are urinating: Slowly tighten the muscles of your pelvic floor until you stop the flow of urine. To perform your daily Kegels, contract these same muscles while sitting, standing, or lying down. Hold for 10 seconds, then release. Repeat 10 to 15 times.

- Avoid getting constipated. Eat plenty of fruits, vegetables, and whole grains.

How Will Being Incontinent Change My Life?

Being incontinent can disrupt your life. It may lead to embarrassing moments, which could eventually cause you to be afraid to leave home. If you withdraw from social activities, your relationships with your friends and family could suffer. You could become depressed, even despondent. Incontinence can also lead to painful skin rashes that might cause you to cut back on your activities. And it can interfere with your sex life. Fortunately, this can all be avoided. If you are experiencing a loss of bladder control, don't try to ignore or hide the problem. See your physician right away. Chances are good that your incontinence is treatable. You may soon be back to your normal routine, doing the things you like.

Varicose Veins

VARICOSE veins are bulging, bluish veins that appear just under the skin. They can show up anywhere on the body but usually are found in the legs and thighs. Varicose veins often ache and sometimes itch. They can also cause swelling and pain in the feet and ankles. In severe cases the veins can rupture, creating open sores on the skin.

Small, weblike clusters of short, thin veins—known as *spider veins*—can also appear on the skin's surface. Spider veins typically appear on the thighs, ankles, and feet. They may also appear on the face.

Both varicose and spider veins are very common, especially among women. Many people also develop **hemorrhoids**, which are varicose veins of the anus.

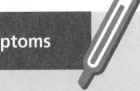

Symptoms

- Bulging, dark blue or purple veins, especially in the legs and thighs
- Swollen, aching legs
- Itching around affected veins
- Discolored skin; sometimes peeling

Causes

Varicose and spider veins form when blood fails to circulate properly, enlarging the veins with pools of blood. The precise cause of this problem is not completely understood, but several factors appear to increase the risk. Age is one important factor, because our veins tend to weaken as we grow older. Being overweight and standing for long periods of time also increase the likelihood of developing varicose and spider veins.

Treatment

Treatment is not always necessary for varicose and spider veins. If the veins are causing you discomfort, however, you should see your physician. He or she will

When to Seek Help

• If you experience aching, pain, and swelling throughout the entire limb	▶ *Seek emergency care immediately.*
• If your toes appear bluish	▶ *Seek emergency care immediately.*
• If you cut a varicose vein, control the bleeding, then	▶ *Call your nurse information service or physician.*
• If you have a vein that is hard, cordlike, and very sensitive to pressure	▶ *Call your nurse information service or physician.*
• If your varicose veins cause discomfort or pain	▶ *Call your nurse information service or physician.*

probably advise you to take regular walks, avoid long periods of standing, and rest with your feet elevated. You may also be advised to wear elastic support stockings. These should be put on first thing in the morning, before blood and fluid have pooled in your feet and ankles. The pain and swelling associated with varicose veins are usually treated with aspirin, ibuprofen, or naproxen.

Several treatments are available for removing varicose and spider veins. Laser surgery is often used to treat small areas of veins, particularly on the face. Another common removal procedure is *sclerotherapy*. This procedure uses a fine needle to inject a solution into the vein that causes it to eventually collapse. Common surgical methods of removing varicose veins include tying off the veins (*ligation*) or pulling them out (*stripping*). These treatments are usually done on large veins. Be sure to discuss all options with your physician before undergoing a particular treatment. Also be aware that new varicose veins can develop in another location after treatment.

At-Home Care

- Avoid standing for long periods of time.

- If you must stand, take frequent breaks. If possible, rest with your feet above chest level.

- Sleep with your legs raised.

- Wear elastic support stockings.

- Avoid sitting with your legs crossed. It can aggravate (but not cause) varicose veins.

Prevention

- Follow the tips under "At-Home Care," above.

- If you are overweight, lose those extra pounds.

- Exercise often.

- Avoid wearing knee-high stockings, tight pantyhose, and garters.

Vision Problems

OUR eyes—and our vision—change as we age. But growing older does not always mean seeing poorly. With proper eye care and regular checkups, many people retain good eyesight into their 80s and beyond.

The three most common eye problems that affect older people are *cataracts, glaucoma,* and *macular degeneration.*

Symptoms

CATARACTS

- Cloudy or blurry vision

- Problems with light—automobile headlights or bright sunlight may seem glaring and uncomfortable

- Seeing halos around lights

- Colors that seem faded

- Poor night vision

- Double or multiple vision (this symptom often goes away as the cataract grows)

- Frequent need to change your eyeglass or contact lens prescription

GLAUCOMA

- Blind spots or loss of peripheral vision

- Sudden and severe eye pain

- Blurred or double vision

- Seeing halos around lights or sensitivity to light, often accompanied by nausea and vomiting

Important: Many people with glaucoma have no symptoms at all.

AGE-RELATED MACULAR DEGENERATION

- Blurred vision, often in only one eye

- Gradual loss of focused, central vision

- Altered perception: Straight lines appear wavy

When to Seek Help

- If you experience sudden loss of vision in one or both eyes ▶ *Seek emergency care immediately.*

- If you experience severe eye pain ▶ *Seek emergency care immediately.*

- If you notice blurry vision, double vision, halos around lights, sensitivity to light, or any other sudden change in your vision ▶ *Call your nurse information service or physician.*

Cataracts

A cataract is an eye disorder in which part or all of the lens, which is usually clear and translucent, becomes cloudy. This causes eyesight to become blurry. Cataracts often develop slowly, over many years. Most people don't notice the problem until it begins to interfere with everyday activities, such as reading, watching television, or driving. Or they may notice they need frequent changes in the prescription of their eyeglasses or contact lenses. More than half of all people aged 65 and older have a cataract.

Causes

Scientists are not sure exactly what causes cataracts to develop. Several factors can increase the risk, however, including smoking and excessive exposure to sunlight. People with **diabetes** are also at greater risk. Eye injuries and infections can cause or worsen the disorder. Cataracts are also sometimes linked to steroid use.

Treatment

Surgery is currently the only corrective treatment for cataracts. During the surgery the clouded lens is removed. It is usually replaced with a clear, plastic lens.

Cataract surgery is very safe. It is generally done right in the surgeon's office or in an outpatient surgical center, and you can return home the same day.

Glaucoma

Glaucoma is a condition in which nerve fibers in the eye become damaged, causing severe vision loss or blindness. It usually begins to develop in middle age and is one of the most common eye problems in people over age 60.

Glaucoma often can be controlled—and blindness prevented—if the condition is detected and treated early. Most people with glaucoma, however, experience no pain or early symptoms. That's why it's important to have your eyes checked regularly.

Causes

Glaucoma is caused by too much fluid pressure inside the eye. The precise reason for this fluid buildup is unknown. African Americans and people with **coronary heart disease** or **diabetes** are at greater risk for developing glaucoma. So are people who are nearsighted. A number of medications, including some for **depression** and asthma, can cause glaucoma. And the condition has been found to run in families.

Treatment

Glaucoma is usually treated with eyedrops or medications that lower pressure in the eye. Surgery is also an option if other treatments fail.

Age-Related Macular Degeneration

Age-related macular degeneration (AMD) is an eye disease that affects central vision. It involves the *macula*, a small area in the retina, the light-sensitive layer of tissue at the back of the eye. The macula is needed for all activities that require focused, straight-ahead vision, such as reading and driving. With age, the macula gradually degenerates. In some cases it degenerates completely, causing a total loss of central vision.

Symptoms of AMD do not usually appear until after age 55. The disease often strikes only one eye at first. Later the other eye may develop symptoms. Physicians have no way of telling, however, if or when the second eye will be affected.

COMMON EYE COMPLAINTS

• *Presbyopia* is the slow loss of the ability to focus on close objects or to see small print. It typically occurs after age 40—when people suddenly find themselves holding reading materials at arm's length. Presbyopia can be corrected with reading glasses.

• *Floaters* are tiny spots or flecks that float across the field of vision. They are harmless but may indicate a more serious eye problem, especially if they occur with light flashes. See your eye doctor if you notice a sudden change in the type or number of spots.

• *Dry* eyes happen when the tear glands produce too few tears. Itching, burning, or even reduced vision may result. See your eye doctor, who can prescribe special eyedrops to relieve the problem. Surgery is sometimes required for more serious cases.

• *Excessive tearing* may be a sign of increased sensitivity to light, wind, or temperature changes. Protecting your eyes (by wearing sunglasses, for instance) may solve the problem. Tearing can also indicate a more serious eye problem, such as an eye infection or a blocked tear duct. See your eye doctor, who can treat or correct both of these conditions.

Source: National Institute on Aging

Causes

AMD usually occurs when new, weak blood vessels grow beneath the macula. Blood and fluid leaks from these vessels, damaging the macula's light-sensitive cells. The risk for getting the disease increases with age. People in their 50s have a 2 percent chance of getting AMD; the risk increases to almost 30 percent for people over age 75. Women appear to be at greater risk than men. So are people who smoke or have high cholesterol. Having a family history of AMD may also increase the risk.

Treatment

AMD can sometimes be treated with laser surgery. The treatment involves aiming a high-energy beam of light directly onto the leaking blood vessels to destroy them.

Prevention

- Have regular health checkups. Many treatable diseases, such as **high blood pressure** and **diabetes**, can cause eye problems.

- Have a complete eye exam every two to three years after age 50 and every year after age 65. If you have **diabetes**, **high blood pressure**, or a family history of eye disease, you may need to have your eyes checked more frequently. Remember: Many eye disorders have no early noticeable symptoms.

- Don't smoke, and avoid smoky areas.

- Wear sunglasses to protect your eyes from the harmful rays of the sun. That includes reflected rays, such as when boating or sitting by a pool.

- Eat plenty of carrots, yellow squash, spinach, collard greens, and other foods rich in the *carotenoids* beta-carotene, lycopene, and lutein (see p. 6). Researchers have found that these yellow to red pigments may offer some protection against age-related macular degeneration.

How Will Having a Vision Problem Change My Life?

Adjusting to a vision loss can be a trying and emotional experience. Many people first feel denial or disbelief, followed by anger and **depression**. Such feelings are normal reactions to the **grief** that comes with adjusting to a major physical change. People with vision problems may also withdraw from former social activities, which may deepen their feelings of loss and isolation. Not being able to drive a car anymore can be a major life adjustment.

If you are having difficulty coping with your vision loss, you may benefit from talking with a psychologist or other qualified counselor. You may also want to consider joining a support group for people who are going through a similar experience. Ask your physician for referrals, or contact the organizations listed in the "Resources" section of this book.

VISION AIDS

Many people with vision problems can be helped with low-vision aids.

• Magnifiers are a great aid for reading. Some are designed to be handheld; others rest directly on reading material. Both types can be bought with a built-in light source. You can also purchase special magnifying glasses, which are stronger than ordinary glasses. They keep your hands free. But you will have to hold reading material closer than with a hand magnifier.

• Telescopes and telescopic glasses can help you see distant objects, such as street signs, television, or a performance in a theater.

• Closed-circuit televisions (CCTVs) help enlarge images on the TV screen. They also allow you to control light and contrast. You can purchase CCTVs that hook up directly to an existing television, or you can buy a separate unit with its own monitor.

• Large-print reading materials include large-print books, newspapers, and magazines. Most bookstores and libraries have special large-print sections. You can also purchase large-print address books, calendars, games and playing cards, and watches. Ask your eye doctor for the names of organizations that sell these and other low-vision aids.

Just for Women

You'll find diseases and health conditions that affect only women on the following pages. These are the illnesses that affect the female reproductive system—**uterine problems** and cancers of the cervix, uterus, and ovaries. **Breast cancer** is included here as well because it is mainly considered a "women's disease," although men can get it, too.

Although **menopause** is not an illness, but a healthy, normal life passage, it is also discussed on these pages. Some of the signs of **menopause**—hot flashes, irregular bleeding, vaginal dryness—can be discomforting. And the decline in hormones that occurs with **menopause** can lead to health problems in some women. Knowing what you can do to ease the discomfort of **menopause** and its possible health consequences can influence your well-being now and in later years.

As a woman, you should also be aware of how the biological and physiological differences between women and men sometimes put women at greater risk for certain illnesses. Understanding those differences may help you make better health decisions. Here are some facts you should know:

- Women who smoke are 20 to 70 percent more likely to develop lung **cancer** than men who smoke the same amount of cigarettes.

- Women are more likely than men to suffer a second heart attack within one year of their first heart attack.

- Women are more likely to get autoimmune diseases (ones in which the body attacks its own tissues), such as rheumatoid **arthritis**, lupus, and multiple sclerosis.

- Women are two to three times more likely to experience **depression** than men. A main reason for this is because women's brains make less of the hormone serotonin.

- Women who have sex with an unprotected partner are two times more likely than men to contract a **sexually transmitted disease**. They are 10 times more likely to contract **HIV**.

- Women over the age of 50 lose more bone than men. That's why 80 percent of people with **osteoporosis** are women.

Menopause

MENOPAUSE is the point in a woman's life when menstruation stops permanently. It generally happens between the ages of 48 and 52, although some women experience an end to menstruation at an earlier or later age. The process is usually gradual, beginning three to five years before the final menstrual period. This transitional phase is called the *climacteric*, or sometimes *perimenopause*. In popular parlance it's known as "the change of life." Menopause is considered complete when a woman has not had a menstrual period for an entire year.

Causes

Menopause occurs when a woman's body stops producing enough of the hormones estrogen and progesterone. As a result, the ovaries stop releasing eggs and menstruation ends. Just what triggers this decline in hormones is not completely understood. But it appears to be governed by our bodies' internal biological clocks. Surgical menopause occurs when a woman's ovaries are removed, often accompanying a complete hysterectomy.

Treatment

Menopause is not an illness. But the decline in hormones that occurs with menopause can lead to health problems in some women. These problems include **osteoporosis**, **coronary heart disease**, and **bladder and other urinary tract infections**. For these reasons, many physicians prescribe replacement hormones (estrogen or a combination of

Symptoms

- Hot flashes—a sudden, often intense feeling of heat; may include sweating

- Night sweats; difficulty sleeping

- Irritability

- Irregular periods

- Vaginal dryness

- Pain during sexual intercourse

When to Seek Help

- If you have irregular or perhaps heavier than normal menstrual periods

  ▶ *Call your nurse information service or physician.*

- If you have bleeding more than six months after your periods stopped

  ▶ *Call your nurse information service or physician.*

- If any of the symptoms of menopause (opposite) bother you

  ▶ *Call your nurse information service or physician.*

estrogen and progesterone) before and after menopause. This treatment is known as *hormone replacement therapy (HRT)*. Physicians also prescribe these drugs to relieve hot flashes and vaginal dryness. HRT has its risks, however. (See "Know the Benefits and Risks of Hormone Replacement Therapy," pp. 210-211.) Be sure to discuss the risks as well as the benefits of HRT with your physician.

If you decide against HRT, you can take many other steps to ease the discomfort of hot flashes, vaginal dryness, and other menopausal changes. And making healthful lifestyle choices can help protect you against **osteoporosis, coronary heart disease**, and other health problems associated with age and declining hormones. (See "Tips for Coping with Hot Flashes" and "At-Home Care," p. 212.)

Common Signs of Menopause

The "symptoms" of menopause are signs of a very natural process. The most common sign is known as *hot flashes*. Women often describe these as sudden flushes of warmth that extend from the chest to the neck and face. A hot flash may last from a few seconds to a few minutes. It may be accompanied by redness of the face and sweating. About 75 to 85 percent of women in the United States report having hot flashes as they pass through menopause. The strength and frequency of the flashes varies from woman to woman. Hot flashes may start several years before menopause. They usually end within two years of the final menstrual period. But some women continue to experience hot flashes into their 60s.

Hot flashes that occur at night are called *night sweats*. Like daytime hot flashes, these can be mild or severe. If severe, night sweats may cause you to awaken in a pool of perspiration. This interruption of sleep can lead to daytime fatigue and sleepiness. Some experts believe that night sweats are also responsible for the **sleep problems** and irritability that some women have during their menopausal years.

Irregular menstrual periods are another common sign of menopause. Your periods may become more frequent—or more spread apart. They may become longer—or shorter. You may also experience a menstrual flow that is heavier—or lighter—than what you have experienced in the past. Or you may skip periods altogether. Irregular periods are quite normal. But you should call your physician if your periods last exceptionally long and/or the bleeding is very heavy. And remember that women over 50 can sometimes become pregnant.

Vaginal dryness is another sign of menopause. Most women notice this change only when having sex. After menopause the vagina takes longer to become lubricated during sexual arousal. For some women this can result in pain during sexual intercourse. Using a lubricant during sex usually resolves the problem.

Know the Benefits and Risks of Hormone Replacement Therapy

Almost every woman eventually needs to make the choice about whether to take hormone replacement therapy (HRT). And if you do choose to take the hormones, for how long should you take them? HRT offers benefits to many women. But it also has its risks. Be sure you discuss all the risks, benefits, and side effects of HRT with your physician before making a decision.

Benefits of HRT

HRT can help ease the hot flashes and related sleep disturbances of menopause. It can also decrease vaginal dryness and discomfort. It does this by increasing the thickness, elasticity, and lubricating ability of vaginal tissue. HRT can also increase the thickness and elasticity of urinary tract tissue. This reduces the risk for developing **bladder and other urinary tract infections** and stress **urinary incontinence**.

HRT can also prevent or greatly reduce bone loss after menopause. This helps protect against **osteoporosis**. It may reduce the incidence of hip fractures. Some studies indicate that women receive this benefit only if HRT is begun within the first few years after menopause. Other studies have shown that HRT can help suppress bone loss even if begun well past menopause. But you must continue to take HRT for it to be effective against bone loss. As soon as you stop taking the hormones, you will lose bone in the same amounts and at the same speed as if you had never taken them.

HRT has been shown to have an effect on *lipoproteins*, the cholesterol compounds that carry fat through the blood. HRT appears to raise the "good" lipoproteins (HDLs) and to lower the "bad" ones (LDLs). Some studies have suggested that this may reduce the risk for **coronary heart disease** and **stroke**, but more recent studies have not found such an effect.

A few preliminary studies indicate that HRT may reduce the risk for developing **Alzheimer's disease**. But scientists caution that much more research needs to be done.

Risks of HRT

Women who have their uterus and take estrogen alone are at increased risk for developing **cancer** of the endometrium (lining of the uterus). Physicians now usually prescribe estrogen with a progestin, a synthetic form of progesterone, for women who still have their uterus. This treatment greatly reduces the risk for endometrial cancer. (A woman whose uterus was removed during a hysterectomy does not need to take progestin.)

Some studies have shown a moderately increased risk for **breast cancer** in women who take HRT for more than five years. The risk is there for women who take an estrogen/progestin combination as well as for those who take estrogen alone.

Women who take HRT are more likely than other women to experience abnormal vaginal bleeding, especially when first starting HRT. As a result, they are more likely to have a *D and C* (*dilation and curettage*) procedure to determine the cause of the bleeding.

HRT also increases the risk for developing **phlebitis**. If you have a history of **phlebitis**, be sure to discuss it with your physician before taking HRT.

Tips for Coping with Hot Flashes

- Stop smoking. Smoking constricts blood vessels, which can make hot flashes more intense.

- Avoid substances that may trigger hot flashes, such as caffeine, alcohol, and spicy foods.

- Keep in shape. Women who exercise and stay in shape tend to report less discomfort with hot flashes.

- Wear cotton and other natural fabrics that "breathe." Also, dress in layers so you can cool down.

- Carry a small battery-run fan in your purse. Pull it out whenever a hot flash hits.

- Keep a thermos of ice water nearby. Sip from it when you feel a hot flash starting.

- Keep a sense of humor about your hot flashes. Talking and laughing about them with friends can be the best coping strategy of all.

At-Home Care

- To strengthen your bones, try to get 1,500 mg of calcium a day in your diet. If you can't get enough calcium from foods, talk to your physician about taking a calcium supplement.

- Make sure you get enough vitamin D. Your body needs it to absorb calcium. You can get enough vitamin D by being outdoors for a short period of time each day. Or drink vitamin D-fortified milk. You may even need a multivitamin supplement.

- Add soy foods, such as tofu and soy milk, to your diet. Soy contains hormonelike chemicals called *phytoestrogens*. Eating soy foods regularly may lower your cholesterol and help protect against **breast cancer**.

- Exercise. It helps your heart, your bones, your mood—just about every aspect of your physical and mental well-being.

- For vaginal dryness, use a lubricant.

- Take time to relax every day. Choose a method of relaxation that you enjoy. It can be a traditional relaxation technique such as yoga or meditation. Or it can be something as simple as setting aside quiet time to read or listen to music.

How Will Going Through Menopause Change My Life?

Most women look upon menopause as a positive life change. They welcome the end of menstruation and experience a new energy and vitality—what anthropologist Margaret Mead called "postmenopausal zest." Many women experience few symptoms or do not find them debilitating. If your mother sailed through menopause, you will likely do so, too.

For some women, however, the "change of life" can be a period of sadness as they recognize that their childbearing years are over. These feelings may be made stronger by other major life changes occurring at the same time—the death of a parent, for example, or children leaving home.

It's important to remember that **depression** is not a sign of menopause. Studies have consistently shown no increase of **depression** among women during their menopausal years. The research is clear: Declining levels of estrogen do not cause **depression**. So going on hormone replacement therapy will not cure it.

If you are experiencing feelings of sadness or **depression** as you pass through menopause, you should consider talking with a psychologist or other qualified counselor. Contact your local mental health association or your physician for a referral. You may also benefit from joining a menopause support group. Many women have found such groups helpful, informative—and fun. To find a support group near you, ask your physician or call your local hospital.

Uterine Problems

THE *uterus* (sometimes called the womb) is a hollow, pear-shaped organ located in the lower abdomen, behind the bladder and in front of the rectum. The narrow, lower end of the uterus is the *cervix*. It leads to the *vagina*. Attached on either side of the uterus at the top are the *fallopian tubes* and *ovaries*.

Each month, during a woman's menstruating years, the lining of the uterus— the *endometrium*—grows and thickens in anticipation of receiving a fertilized egg. If an egg does not become fertilized and an embryo is not formed, the endometrium is shed through the vagina, along with some blood. This process is known, of course, as *menstruation*. For most women menstruation ends around age 50, with **menopause**.

Symptoms

FIBROIDS

- Heavy or irregular menstrual bleeding
- Pain in the lower abdomen or back
- A feeling of fullness in the lower abdomen
- Frequent urination
- Pain during sexual intercourse

Important: Many women with fibroids have no symptoms at all.

PROLAPSED UTERUS

- Urine leakage
- Difficulty urinating or moving bowels
- A feeling of fullness or pressure in the lower abdomen
- Pain in the lower back

DYSFUNCTIONAL UTERINE BLEEDING (DUB)

- Heavy, irregular, or constant premenopausal bleeding

When to Seek Help

- If you feel a sharp or chronic pain in your lower abdomen

  ▶ *Call your nurse information service or physician immediately.*

- If your menstrual periods are very heavy for a long time

  ▶ *Call your nurse information service or physician.*

- If you have bleeding more than six months after your menstrual periods have stopped

  ▶ *Call your nurse information service or physician.*

Many problems can affect the uterus, both before and after **menopause**. Three of the most common noncancerous uterine problems are fibroids, prolapsed uterus, and dysfunctional uterine bleeding (DUB). For a discussion of (endometrial) uterine cancer, see pp. 224-225.

Fibroids

Fibroids, or *leiomyomas*, are noncancerous tumors that grow in the muscular wall of the uterus. They vary in size and may grow quickly or slowly. Sometimes they cause pain or bleeding. But often fibroids cause no symptoms at all and are discovered only during a routine pelvic exam (an internal examination of the reproductive organs) in a physician's office.

Heavy bleeding in menstruating women is the most common symptom of fibroids. It is also the most worrisome, as it can lead to *anemia*, or low levels of iron in the blood. In addition, fibroids can sometimes press on the bladder or rectum. This can result in frequent urination or **constipation**. Fibroids can also make sexual intercourse painful.

Fibroids are very common. About one-quarter to one-half of all women will eventually develop them.

Causes

The cause of fibroids is unknown. But their growth appears linked to the hormone estrogen. Fibroids tend to grow during pregnancy, when a woman's estrogen levels are high. Taking birth control pills and hormone replacement therapy for **menopause** can also cause fibroids to enlarge. But fibroids tend to shrink after a woman passes through **menopause** and her estrogen levels drop.

Treatment

When a fibroid is causing no symptoms, "watchful waiting" may be the best treatment. This is especially true for women who are approaching **menopause**. Most fibroids shrink after menstruation finally ends. If you take this wait-and-see approach, you will need to visit your physician periodically to monitor the growth of the fibroid.

If you are experiencing occasional pelvic pain or discomfort, your physician may prescribe an over-the-counter pain reliever or an anti-inflammatory medication. Sometimes *gonadotropin releasing hormone (GnRH) agonists* are prescribed to shrink fibroids. But these drugs can increase the risk for developing **osteoporosis** if taken for more than six months, and once the use of the drug has stopped, the fibroids usually return.

Years ago the standard treatment for fibroids was a *hysterectomy*, or surgical removal of the entire uterus. But today there are newer, less invasive surgical treatments. One of these is *myomectomy*, a procedure that uses lasers (high-intensity lights) to remove the fibroid while leaving the uterus intact. In addition, some fibroids can be destroyed by freezing or burning them or by cutting off their blood supply in a procedure called *embolization*.

Prolapsed Uterus

A *prolapsed uterus* is a uterus that has tilted or slipped. In severe cases the uterus can slip so far down that it actually hangs out of the vagina. A prolapsed uterus can cause feelings of pressure and discomfort in the abdomen. It can also lead to **urinary incontinence**.

Causes

A prolapsed uterus happens when the ligaments that hold the uterus to the wall of the pelvis weaken. The uterus then slides downward. The weakening of the ligaments often begins during childbirth. Women who have had babies who weighed more than 8 pounds at birth are at increased risk. The ligaments may repair themselves over time, but they may never return to their former strength. Later, with age, the ligaments may weaken further. Being overweight can contribute to the problem.

Treatment

A prolapsed uterus cannot repair itself. If you have any symptoms of this problem, see your physician. In mild cases doing exercises that strengthen the muscles supporting the uterus may be the only treatment needed. These exercises, known as Kegels, should be done daily. (See "At-Home Care," p. 219.)

Taking estrogen can sometimes keep the muscles and tissues that support the uterus from weakening further. Your physician may also recommend that you try a *pessary*. This rubber device is inserted into the vagina to hold the uterus in place. It has several drawbacks. It may cause irritation, may interfere with sexual intercourse, and must be taken out regularly by a physician for cleaning.

In severe cases surgery may be required. One type of surgery tightens the weakened muscles without removing the uterus. But if the uterus has dropped so far that it is coming through the vagina, a hysterectomy may be needed. This surgery is sometimes done through the vagina, without opening the abdomen.

Dysfunctional Uterine Bleeding (DUB)

Dysfunctional uterine bleeding (DUB) is irregular, heavy, or constant bleeding from the uterus. It often affects women as they approach and pass through **menopause**. It is the result of a hormone imbalance in the body. DUB is *not* caused by a specific condition or disease, such as uterine fibroids or **cancer** (although those disorders can result in uterine bleeding).

Causes

Many factors can trigger the hormonal imbalance that causes DUB. For women approaching **menopause**, DUB is usually caused by a lack of ovulation, or failure of eggs to be released from the ovaries. When a woman does not ovulate, her ovaries do not produce the hormone progesterone. Without progesterone the lining of the uterus keeps growing. When it finally does break down, it sheds very heavily. It may also shed incompletely or irregularly.

Treatment

Your physician will first want to rule out any medical conditions that may be causing the abnormal bleeding. You will be given a pelvic exam and perhaps a blood test to determine the levels of hormones in your body. Your physician may also suggest other tests, such as an *endometrial biopsy* or a D and C (dilation and curettage), both of which involve removing a small sample of uterine tissue for examination under a microscope.

If tests show that the abnormal bleeding is caused by a hormonal imbalance and not by an underlying medical condition, there are several possible avenues of treatment. Your physician may recommend that the bleeding be watched and monitored for a few months to see if it stops on its own. During this time you may be advised to take iron supplements as a precaution against anemia.

Your physician may prescribe progesterone or some other form of hormone therapy to help control the bleeding. In severe cases a *hysterectomy*, or surgical removal of the uterus, is sometimes recommended. A newer, less invasive procedure called *endometrial ablation* is now often used in place of a hysterectomy. This procedure controls bleeding by destroying the endometrium with lasers. Another new nonsurgical procedure, called *uterine balloon therapy*, uses a balloon to deliver heat to the lining of the uterus, destroying the lining and reducing bleeding.

When Is a Hysterectomy Necessary?

By age 60 one of four American women will have had a *hysterectomy*, or surgery to remove their uterus. Some medical experts say hysterectomies are done too often in the United States. They point out that other safer, less invasive treatments are now available for most women with noncancerous uterine problems.

When is a hysterectomy necessary? That depends on many factors, including a woman's age, her symptoms, and the seriousness of her condition. A hysterectomy is standard—and lifesaving—treatment for **cancer** of the cervix or uterus. But for noncancerous uterine problems a hysterectomy is usually needed only in extreme situations.

You should always discuss with your physician all your treatment options before undergoing a hysterectomy. Also, get a second—and possibly a third—opinion from other physicians. You may also want to contact some of the organizations listed in the "Resources" section of this book.

At-Home Care

- Practice Kegel exercises daily. These exercises strengthen the muscles that control the flow of urine. You can identify the muscles you need to exercise while you are urinating: Slowly tighten the muscles of your pelvic floor until you stop the flow of urine. To perform your daily Kegels, contract these same muscles while sitting, standing, or lying down. Hold for 10 seconds, then release. Repeat 10 to 15 times.

- For occasional pelvic pain or discomfort associated with fibroids, take an over-the-counter pain reliever. You can also try lessening the discomfort by placing a hot-water bottle or hot pack on your lower abdomen.

- Eat less red meat—and more green vegetables and fruit. Recent research indicates that women with fibroids tend to have eaten more ham, beef, and other red meat. They also have eaten fewer daily servings of green vegetables and fruits.

How Will Having a Hysterectomy Change My Life?

How you feel after a hysterectomy may depend on how you felt before the surgery. Women who have the operation to relieve the pain or discomfort of a severe uterine problem often report feeling relieved after their hysterectomy. Many also experience a renewed sense of energy.

In fact, research has shown that women do not have a higher rate of **depression** after a hysterectomy than before. Nor is it true that women generally experience a loss in libido after a hysterectomy. If your sex life was good before the operation, it will probably continue to be.

Some women, however, do become depressed or lose interest in sex after their hysterectomy. If you are experiencing these feelings, you may benefit from talking with a psychologist or other qualified counselor. Contact your local mental health association or ask your physician for a referral.

Women's Cancers: Breast, Cervical, Endometrial, and Ovarian

Breast Cancer

After skin **cancer**, breast cancer is the most common type of **cancer** diagnosed in women in the United States. Each year more than 175,000 American women learn they have breast cancer. Two of every three of those women are over age 50.

The two main types of breast cancer are *lobular* and *ductal carcinomas*. Lobular carcinomas develop in the *lobules*, the small sacs that produce milk. Ductal carcinomas begin in the lining of the ducts that carry milk to the nipple.

Breast cancers do not all grow and spread at the same rate. Some take years to spread beyond the breast; others do so quickly. Cancer cells that spread beyond the breast are often found in the lymph nodes under the arm. When the cells reach these nodes, they may have traveled to other parts of the body, such as the bones, liver, or lungs. Breast cancer that has spread beyond the breast is called *metastatic breast cancer*.

Fortunately, breast cancer is often treatable if caught early. That's why it's so important to get regular mammograms after age 50. But even breast cancer that has spread can often be controlled successfully for years.

Causes

Scientists are not sure exactly what causes **cancer** to develop in breast tissue. But they have identified some major risk factors. These include having the following:

- A personal history of an earlier breast cancer

- A mother, sister, daughter, or two or more close relatives, such as cousins, with a history of breast cancer (especially if the **cancer** was diagnosed at a young age)

- A specific defective gene—BRCA1 or BRCA2—that is known to make women more susceptible to breast cancer

- A diagnosis of atypical hyperplasia or other breast condition that may predispose a woman to breast cancer

- A history of two or more breast biopsies for benign breast disease

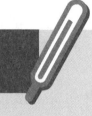

Symptoms

BREAST CANCER

- A lump or thickening in or near the breast or in the underarm area

- A change in the size or shape of the breast

- A discharge from the nipple

- A change in the color or feel of the skin of the breast, areola, or nipple (dimpled, puckered, or scaly)

CERVICAL CANCER

- An unusual discharge from the vagina

- Vaginal bleeding after sexual intercourse

- Pain during sexual intercourse

- Vaginal bleeding more than six months after **menopause**

Important: Early cervical cancer usually has no symptoms.

ENDOMETRIAL CANCER

- Unusual vaginal bleeding or discharge, particularly after **menopause**

- Pain in the lower abdomen

- Unexplained weight loss

- Vaginal bleeding more than six months after **menopause**

OVARIAN CANCER

- Feelings of fullness or bloating in the abdomen

- Digestive problems, including gas, diarrhea, **constipation**, or **indigestion**

- Loss of appetite

- Frequent need to urinate

- Unusual vaginal bleeding

Important: In its early stages, ovarian cancer often has no symptoms.

When to Seek Help

- If you notice any lumps or changes in the appearance, color, or feel of your breasts ▶ *Call your nurse information service or physician.*

- If you have a discharge from one of your nipples ▶ *Call your nurse information service or physician.*

- If you have any unusual discharge from your vagina ▶ *Call your nurse information service or physician.*

- If you experience any abnormal bleeding ▶ *Call your nurse information service or physician.*

- If you experience bleeding or pain during sexual intercourse ▶ *Call your nurse information service or physician.*

- If you have bleeding more than six months after your menstrual periods have stopped ▶ *Call your nurse information service or physician.*

Other factors may also increase a woman's risk for developing breast cancer. They include the following:

- Exposure to intensive radiation therapy for treatment of other forms of **cancer** or tuberculosis

- Use of hormone replacement therapy after menopause

An important fact to keep in mind: Most women considered at high risk never develop breast cancer. And many with no risk factors get the disease.

Treatment

Treatment will depend on the type, size, location, and stage (extent) of the tumor in the breast. A woman's age, general health, and feelings about treatment options are also usually considered.

Local treatments, such as surgery and radiation, are used to remove, destroy, or control the cancer cells in a specific area. Systemic treatments, such as chemotherapy and hormonal therapy, are used to destroy or control cancer cells that have spread to other areas of the body. Your physician may recommend one form of treatment or a combination.

Choosing a treatment is a complex issue. Discuss your options in detail with your physician. You should also seek a second—and possibly a third—opinion from other physicians.

Cervical Cancer

Cervical cancer begins in the lining of the cervix, the lower part of the uterus. This **cancer** takes many years to develop. First, some cells change from normal to precancerous. This phase is called *dysplasia*. It occurs most often in women between the ages of 25 and 35.

Sometimes the precancerous changes go away without any treatment. When the cells turn cancerous they enter a phase called *carcinoma in situ*. Women between the ages of 30 and 40 are most likely to be diagnosed with this stage of cervical cancer.

The cancerous cells may then spread to nearby tissue. If the cells enter the bloodstream or lymphatic system, they can travel to even more distant organs. This invasive form of cervical cancer is found most often in women over the age of 40.

Cervical cancer, therefore, is a serious health concern for older women. About 41 percent of the 4,800 cervical cancer deaths that occur each year in the United States are in women over the age of 65.

Fortunately, when found and treated early, cervical cancer is highly curable. Unfortunately, many older women underestimate their risk and do not have regular Pap tests—screenings that can help detect the **cancer**. All sexually active women under age 70 who have not had a hysterectomy should have a Pap test at least every three years. Women 70 or older should discuss with their physician how often to be tested.

Causes

Scientists have identified several risk factors for cervical cancer:

- HPV (human papillomavirus) infection. This **sexually transmitted disease** has been linked to cervical cancer. Not every woman who has been infected with HPV develops the **cancer**, however.

- **HIV** infection (the virus that causes **AIDS**). Because women with HIV often have weakened immune systems, they are more vulnerable to developing an HPV infection and cervical cancer.

- Smoking. Chemicals produced by smoking may damage the DNA in cells of the cervix. This increases the chances of **cancer** developing.

Treatment

Treatment for cervical cancer depends largely on the stage of the disease or how far it has spread. Your age and your general health may also influence the choice of treatment.

Early changes that show up in a Pap test may not need immediate treatment. Some precancerous conditions go away on their own and may therefore require only careful monitoring by your physician. Severe dysplasia and later stages of cervical cancer are usually treated surgically, chemically (chemotherapy), or with radiation. Sometimes a combination of treatments is used. Discuss your treatment options with your physician. You should also seek a second—and possibly a third—opinion from other physicians.

Endometrial Cancer

Endometrial cancer is **cancer** that begins in the *endometrium,* the inner lining of the uterus. It tends to be a slow-growing **cancer** and generally is found before it has spread very far. Most women diagnosed with endometrial cancer are over age 50.

Causes

Many of the known risk factors for endometrial cancer are linked to the balance in the body between the hormones estrogen and progesterone. Estrogen stimulates cell division in the endometrium; progesterone opposes it. A high level of cell division means a greater chance of a cell mutating into **cancer**. So the longer the endometrium is exposed to estrogen—and unopposed by progesterone—the greater the risk for developing this **cancer**.

The risk factors for endometrial cancer include the following:

- Early menarche (starting menstruation before age 12).

- Late **menopause** (after age 52).

- A history of infertility.

- Never having given birth.

- Obesity. Fat tissue can produce estrogen, increasing a women's exposure to the hormone.

Did You Know?

The breast cancer death rate has been going down in recent years. Scientists think the drop is because more women are having mammograms. With early screening, breast cancer can be caught at a more treatable stage. New, more effective treatments for breast cancer may also be a factor in why women with breast cancer are living longer.

- Taking the drug tamoxifen to treat breast cancer. This small risk is more than balanced, however, by the often lifesaving benefit of taking tamoxifen for breast cancer.

- Hormone replacement therapy. The risk is greatest when estrogen is taken alone, without progesterone. Adding progesterone may diminish the risk, but it doesn't eliminate it. That's because some of the protective effects of the progesterone may be lost if the hormones are taken for more than five years.

- A diet high in animal fat.

- Family history. Endometrial cancer tends to run in families.

- A history of breast or ovarian cancer.

Treatment

Endometrial cancer is usually treated with surgery to take out the uterus and the ovaries. If the disease has spread beyond the uterus, your physician may treat you after surgery with hormones, radiation, or chemotherapy.

Ovarian Cancer

Ovarian cancer begins in the *ovaries*, the almond-shaped organs on either side of the uterus that produce eggs and hormones. This **cancer** can strike at any age, but it is most common after **menopause**.

Ovarian cancer is treatable if found in its earliest stages. But detection is difficult because the disease has few early symptoms. Any symptoms that do appear may be vague. They may be mistaken for other, minor ailments. Often the **cancer** has spread by the time it is diagnosed.

Causes

Several factors increase a woman's risk for getting ovarian cancer. These include the following:

- Age. Most ovarian cancers occur after **menopause**.
- Fertility drugs. Women who have taken the drug clomiphene citrate for prolonged periods to get pregnant are at an increased risk for developing ovarian cancer.
- Reproductive history. Women who started menstruating before age 12, had no children, or had their first child after age 30 are at increased risk. So are women who experienced **menopause** after age 50.
- Family history of ovarian cancer. Most women with ovarian cancer have no family history of the disease. But women with a mother, sister, or daughter who had the disease are at increased risk.
- Breast cancer. Women who have had breast cancer are at increased risk for developing ovarian cancer.

Treatment

The main treatments for ovarian cancer are surgery, chemotherapy, and radiation therapy. In some cases a combination of these treatments is recommended. What treatment is right for you will depend largely on the stage (extent) of your disease. Your age and your general health may also influence the choice of treatment. Discuss your treatment options with your physician. You should also seek a second—and possibly a third—opinion from other physicians.

Prevention

- Have a mammogram every one to two years until age 69. If you are 70 or older, discuss with your physician how often you should have a mammogram.

- Check your breasts once a month. Also, have your breasts examined by your physician every year at your annual checkup.

- If you are sexually active, have a Pap test every one to three years, unless your physician advises differently.

- If you come from a family with a history of ovarian cancer, you may want to consider getting some genetic testing and counseling. Such testing can determine whether you are at high risk for getting the disease. Some physicians recommend that women at very high risk have their ovaries removed as a preventive measure.

- Control your weight.

- Eat a low-fat diet. Make sure your meals include plenty of green leafy vegetables, fruits, and whole grains.

How to Do a Breast Self-Exam

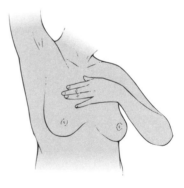

By doing a simple breast self-exam every month, you may increase your chances of finding breast cancer early. Breast cancer usually can be cured if you find it early.

To detect a lump, press firmly with the pads of your fingers. Move your *left* hand over your *right* breast in a circle, beginning at the nipple and moving out. Now check your *left* breast with your *right* hand in the same way. Be sure to check your armpit, too.

Look in the mirror also to detect changes in the appearance of your breasts. If there is any swelling, dimpling, redness, discharge from the nipple, or other change, tell your doctor right away. Remember, a breast self-exam is not a substitute for a mammogram and breast exam by your physician.

Just for Men

You will find diseases and health conditions that affect only men on the following pages. These are the illnesses that concern the male reproductive system—**prostate problems** and cancers of the prostate and testes. It's important that men learn how to recognize the early signs of these health problems as most can be successfully treated if caught early.

Unfortunately, many men ignore early signs of illness. They tend to avoid calling a doctor until their symptoms have become severe. This hesitancy to seek medical care is one of the major reasons men live, on average, about six years less than women. (Currently, average life expectancy for men is 73.1 years; for women, it's 79.1 years.) Women see their doctors a whopping 150 percent more frequently than men. As a result, their health problems are often detected at an earlier, more treatable stage.

If you are a man who has not been in the habit of seeing a doctor regularly, now is the time to make a change. Build a partnership with your physician. (See pp. 43-50 for information on how to do this.) And be sure to stay current with all preventive health screenings (p. 41).

Also, be aware that your gender puts you at higher risk for certain illnesses. Here are some facts you should know:

- Men have much higher rates of lung **cancer**, colorectal **cancer**, and bladder **cancer** than women.

- Men are 13 times more likely than women to die as a result of an on-the-job injury.

- Men are twice as likely to die from skin **cancer** than women.

- Two million men have **osteoporosis** in the United States, including one-third of men over age 75.

- Hip fractures are more serious in men than in women. Men have a 26 percent higher death rate within a year after a hip fracture than women do.

- Men account for only 1 percent of **breast cancer** cases in the United States. But their **cancer** is usually diagnosed at a more advanced stage. This is mainly because they failed to recognize the disease's symptoms in its early stages.

Prostate Problems

THE prostate is a small, walnut-shaped organ that surrounds the *urethra* (the tube that carries urine from the bladder to the end of the penis). It produces most of the fluid in semen. The prostate gland is mainly regulated by the hormone testosterone, which is produced in the testicles.

Prostate problems are very common in men over age 50. Such problems can create both urinary and **sexual problems**. Most prostate problems can be treated successfully, however. The most common noncancerous prostate problems are *benign prostatic hyperplasia (BPH)* and *prostatitis*. (For a discussion of **cancer** of the prostate, see pp. 234-237.)

For most prostate problems, your primary care physician will probably refer you to a *urologist* (a physician who specializes in diseases of the urinary system).

Symptoms

BENIGN PROSTATIC HYPERPLASIA (BPH)

- A weak or interrupted stream of urine

- Dribbling after urination

- An urge to urinate right away

- More frequent urination, especially at night

PROSTATITIS

- Difficulty urinating

- More frequent urination

- Pain in the pelvis and genital area

- Blood in semen or urine

- Painful ejaculations

- Fever and chills (acute prostatitis)

Benign Prostatic Hyperplasia (BPH)

The prostate enlarges with age—a condition known as *benign prostatic hyperplasia (BPH)*. As the gland slowly gets bigger, it pushes against the urethra. This can make it difficult to urinate. It can also lead to a need to pass urine more frequently, especially at night. In rare cases the urethra becomes completely blocked, making it impossible to urinate. This is a very serious condition that requires immediate medical care. Prostate enlargement is common in older men—and as inevitable as wrinkles and gray hair. By their 50s more than half the men in the United States have an enlarged prostate. The percentage jumps to 90 percent for men over 80.

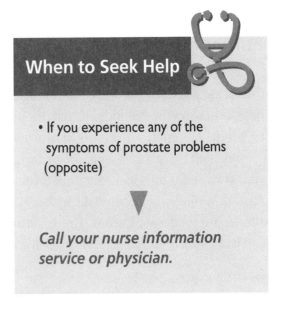

When to Seek Help

- If you experience any of the symptoms of prostate problems (opposite)

▼

Call your nurse information service or physician.

Causes

The cause of BPH is not known. It may be linked to declining levels of the hormone testosterone.

Treatment

BPH is usually detected with a rectal exam. Your physician may also use a *cystoscope*, an instrument that is inserted through the penis, to examine your urethra, prostate, and bladder.

BPH does not need to be treated unless you are bothered by symptoms. If you do require treatment, your physician may prescribe drugs to help shrink the prostate gland. Other drugs can help relax the muscles that are pinching the urethra. This may make it easier to urinate. Sometimes BPH can lead to **urinary tract infections**; in these cases antibiotics are usually prescribed.

Surgery to remove part of the enlarged prostate is generally recommended in severe cases. It is very successful in relieving symptoms but can result in complications. Some men become impotent after the surgery; others may be able to have an erection but become sterile. Several kinds of surgery are available. Be sure to discuss with your physician the risks and benefits of all options of treatment.

Prostatitis

Prostatitis is an infection or inflammation of the prostate gland. The infection causes the prostate to swell, constricting the urethra. Prostatitis can lead to intense pain, urinary complications, sexual dysfunction, and infertility. It strikes men of all ages, but older men with enlarged prostates are more susceptible.

Prostatitis can be either acute or chronic. *Acute prostatitis* usually comes on suddenly. Symptoms include chills, fever, and pain in the lower back and genital area. Urinating may become difficult and painful. *Chronic prostatitis* produces similar but milder symptoms. There is usually no fever, however. Chronic prostatitis can last a long time. It also tends to come back again and again.

Causes

In some cases prostatitis is caused by a bacterial infection. The infection may have spread from the urinary tract. In most cases of prostatitis, however, evidence of disease-causing bacteria cannot be found. Scientists do not know what triggers this nonbacterial form of the disease.

Treatment

Antibiotics are usually used to treat prostatitis. These drug treatments often fail, however, because bacteria do not cause most cases of prostatitis. To help ease urination, your physician may also prescribe drugs to relax the muscles of the prostate gland.

Nonbacterial prostatitis generally goes away by itself. To ease your discomfort, your physician may recommend warm baths and over-the-counter pain relievers. Self-massaging the prostate to release fluids can also help.

At-Home Care

- Unless your physician has limited your fluid intake, drink plenty of water. Dehydration stresses the prostate. But try to avoid fluids after the evening meal. And be sure to empty your bladder before going to bed.

- Avoid caffeine and alcohol. Both can dehydrate the body.

- Try warm baths to relieve pain. Also, try over-the-counter pain relievers.

- Massage the prostate. Your physician can show you how to do this.

- Have a digital rectal exam as part of your annual checkup. Be sure to discuss with your physician any changes in urinary habits or symptoms that may be bothering you.

How Will Having a Prostate Problem Change My Life?

If you have a mild prostate problem, you may not need to change your daily activities. As your symptoms worsen, however, you may find yourself modifying or curtailing much of your daily routine. Men with severe prostate problems often find that they have to stay near a bathroom. They may wear dark pants to hide urine leakage. Because the constant urge to urinate keeps them up at night, they may also feel tired during the day. They may need frequent naps to catch up on lost sleep.

Such adjustments can have a profound effect on your lifestyle. It can also lead to social withdrawal and **depression**. If you are experiencing symptoms of a prostate problem, talk to your physician. Treatment of the problem can help you regain your normal activities.

Men's Cancers: Prostate and Testicular

Prostate Cancer

Prostate cancer is the second most common **cancer** diagnosed in American men, after skin **cancer**. Some 179,000 men are diagnosed with the disease each year.

Prostate cancer is also the second leading cause of **cancer** deaths among men in the United States, after lung cancer. About 37,000 men die of the disease annually. Prostate cancer affects mostly older men. About 80 percent of all cases are diagnosed in men over age 65. The disease has become more common, perhaps because men are living longer.

Symptoms

PROSTATE CANCER

Important: Many men with prostate cancer have no symptoms. As the disease progresses, the following symptoms may appear:

- Difficulty starting or stopping urination
- A weak or interrupted stream of urine
- Dribbling after urination
- A frequent need to urinate
- Painful ejaculation
- Blood in the urine or semen
- Continuing pain in the lower back, pelvis, or upper thighs
- Loss of weight, fatigue, nausea

TESTICULAR CANCER

- A lump in either testicle
- Any enlargement of a testicle
- A feeling of heaviness in the scrotum
- A dull ache in the lower abdomen or the groin
- A sudden collection of fluid in the scrotum
- Pain or discomfort in a testicle or in the scrotum
- Breast enlargement or tenderness

When to Seek Help

• If you experience difficulty or pain while urinating	▶ *Call your nurse information service or physician.*
• If you notice blood in your urine or semen	▶ *Call your nurse information service or physician.*
• If you have chronic pain in your lower back, pelvis, or upper thighs	▶ *Call your nurse information service or physician.*
• If you notice an unusual lump or swelling in a testicle	▶ *Call your nurse information service or physician.*
• If you have any kind of pain or discomfort in the scrotum	▶ *Call your nurse information service or physician.*

Early in the disease, the **cancer** stays in the prostate. In fact, it can remain in this "dormant" stage for years, causing no symptoms. Many men with prostate cancer outlive the disease and die of other, unrelated causes. Often they die not even knowing that they had the **cancer**. But in other men the **cancer** spreads outside the prostate to surrounding areas, including the lymph nodes, pelvic bones, lower back, and spine. Once the **cancer** has spread, it becomes life-threatening.

Causes

Scientists don't know what causes prostate cancer, but the chances of developing it increase with age. Other risk factors include the following:

- Race. African American men are diagnosed with the disease at later stages and die of prostate cancer at higher rates than white men. The incidence of this disease among African American men is the highest in the world.

- Nationality. Prostate cancer is most common in North America and northwestern Europe. It is less common in Asia, Africa, Central America, and South America.

- Diet. Eating a high-fat diet increases the risk for prostate cancer. This may be because men who eat a lot of high-fat foods tend to eat fewer fruits and vegetables and more dairy products. Recent research suggests that a diet high in calcium, which is found in dairy products, also increases the risk.

- Family history. Prostate cancer tends to run in families. This suggests that it may have an inherited or genetic component. Your risk for developing this disease doubles if your father or brother had it.

- Vasectomy. Some studies indicate that men who have had a vasectomy may be at slightly increased risk for developing prostate cancer. Other studies show no increased risk.

Diagnosis and Treatment

Prostate cancer may be found during a routine rectal examination. That's why men with symptoms should have a rectal exam. If you have symptoms or risk factors for prostate cancer, your physician may also recommend that you have a prostate specific antigen (PSA) blood test. (See "The PSA Test: One Tool for Diagnosing Prostate Cancer," opposite.)

If your physician suspects prostate cancer, he or she may recommend a biopsy. During this simple surgical procedure your physician will use a needle to remove small tissue samples from the prostate. The samples are then examined under a microscope. If **cancer** is found, you will be given other tests to determine what type of treatment is needed.

Prostate cancer can be treated in several ways. The choice depends largely on whether or not the **cancer** has spread beyond the prostate. Your age, general health, and feelings about treatment options and their side effects are also considered.

Treatments for prostate cancer include surgery, radiation therapy, hormone therapy, and watchful waiting. Surgery generally involves removing the entire prostate and surrounding tissues—an operation called a radical prostatectomy. In the past, most men who underwent this surgery became impotent. Surgeons are now able to remove the prostate in a way that can preserve the nerves that control penile erections. Many men undergoing a prostatectomy experience **urinary incontinence** after the surgery. The problem usually clears up, however, within a few weeks or months.

THE PSA TEST:
One Tool for Diagnosing Prostate Cancer

The prostate specific antigen (PSA) blood test measures how much of the PSA protein is in your blood. PSA levels tend to be higher in men who have prostate cancer.

But the PSA test is not always accurate. PSA levels are also high in men with other, noncancerous prostate conditions, such as prostatitis (p. 232) and benign prostatic hyperplasia (BPH) (p. 231). Being sexually active within two days of having the test can also cause high PSA readings.

On the other hand, some men with prostate cancer sometimes have low PSA readings. Several medications and herbal preparations are among the factors that can lower readings.

Although it is not always accurate, the PSA test is considered by many to be a valuable tool for the early detection of prostate cancer, especially for people who have symptoms or are at increased risk. Some researchers believe it has helped to dramatically increase the number of prostate cancers found at an early, curable stage. Still, inaccurate PSA readings can lead to unnecessary treatment. Before taking the test, be sure to talk with your physician about its risks as well as its potential benefits.

If your **cancer** is small, slow growing, and not causing symptoms, your physician may recommend watchful waiting. This process involves closely monitoring the **cancer** without treating it. Older men and those with other illnesses sometimes choose this option.

Discuss all your treatment options with your physician. You should also seek a second—and possibly a third—opinion from other physicians.

Testicular Cancer

Testicular cancer is **cancer** that develops in one or both of the *testicles*, or *testes*. The testicles are glands contained within a sac of skin called the *scrotum*, which hangs beneath the penis. These glands make several hormones, including *testosterone*, the hormone that causes such male traits as facial hair and lower voice pitch. They also produce sperm. The testicles usually descend into the scrotum before birth.

Your chances of developing testicular cancer decrease dramatically after age 40. But you can get the disease at any age, so you should be aware of its symptoms. The first warning sign is usually a change in the size or shape of a testicle. You may also notice a firm, often painless, lump. It's important that you become familiar with the size and feeling of your normal testicles so you can notice any changes as soon as they occur. (See "How to Do a Testicular Self-Exam, opposite.)

Compared with other types of **cancer**, testicular cancer is relatively rare. It accounts for only about 1 percent of cancers in men. The other good news about testicular cancer is that it is now one of the most curable of cancers. Because of new advances in treatment, testicular cancer has a cure rate of more than 95 percent when found early.

Causes

The exact cause of testicular cancer is unknown. White men and men whose testicles did not descend by age 3 are at greatest risk. The disease also tends to run in families; your risk for developing this disease increases if your father or brother had it.

Exposure to certain chemicals may also contribute to development of the disease. Some studies have found that testicular cancer occurs more often among men with certain occupations. Miners, oil and gas workers, leather workers, food and beverage processing workers, janitors, and utility workers seem to be particularly at risk.

Injury to the testicles has *not* been shown to cause testicular cancer. Nor does having a vasectomy increase the risk.

Treatment

The first treatment for testicular cancer is removal of the affected testicle. The surgery is necessary because it is the only safe way to know with certainty that **cancer** is present. It's also needed to determine exactly what type of testicular cancer it is. If the **cancer** has spread, your physician may recommend additional surgery and/or chemotherapy or radiation.

How to Do a Testicular Self-Exam

By doing a simple self-examination periodically, you can greatly increase your chances of finding testicular cancer early.

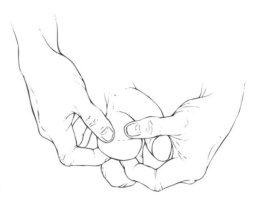

The best time for the self-exam is just after a warm bath or shower. The tissue of your scrotum will be more relaxed. While standing, gently roll each of the testicles between the fingers and thumbs of both hands. Feel for lumps or bumps. If you find any changes, call your physician.

Important: Not all lumps found on the testicle are cancerous. A lump may also be a hernia, a cyst, or even an enlarged blood vessel.

Prevention

- Exercise and maintain a healthy weight. Doing both reduces the risk for prostate cancer.

- Eat foods rich in lycopenes, beta-carotene, and selenium. These antioxidants seem to lower prostate cancer risk. (For a list of which foods contain high amounts of these antioxidants, see p. 6.)

- Add soy foods, such as tofu and soy milk, to your diet. Soy contains isoflavones, which appear to inhibit the growth of prostate cancer cells.

- Take vitamin E. Some studies suggest that taking 50 milligrams of vitamin E daily can lower the risk for developing prostate cancer by one-third.

- Have a digital rectal exam as part of your periodic health exam. Be sure to discuss with your physician any changes in urinary habits or symptoms that may be bothering you.

- Do a testicular self-exam periodically. (See "How to Do a Testicular Self-Exam," above.)

Your Dental Health

At first blush, it looks like bad news: According to the American Dental Association (ADA), older people get more cavities—three times more—than children.

But consider this: One generation ago, the majority of older people lost all their teeth. No teeth, no cavities. So the fact that cavities are no longer just for kids is actually good news. It means that most older people today have retained some or all of their natural teeth.

This teeth-retention trend should continue. Experts say in the next 20 years the number of people over age 65 needing dentures will drop from 30 percent to 10 percent.

In the past, dentures were usually our destiny. Today, we are more hopeful than past generations about our dental health, just as we are more hopeful about our health in general. According to an ADA survey, 64 percent of American adults considered their teeth and oral health to be much or somewhat better than that of their parents when their parents were the same age. We like the idea of keeping our teeth and mouth in good shape, of enjoying a full range of foods, and of keeping our bright smiles.

Aging can bring changes that make your teeth and mouth more vulnerable to cavities and other problems. But with proper care, your teeth can last a lifetime. That should bring a smile to your face.

The key phrase is "with proper care." You can brush up on proper care in the following pages. As you do, remember this traditional dental proverb: *Be true to your teeth or your teeth will be false to you.*

Take Care of Your Teeth and Gums

How many strains of bacteria do you think are in your mouth—10? 20? 100? Would you believe almost 500 and counting? Most of the bacteria are friendly. They help to digest food and ward off attack by less friendly, disease-causing bacteria that can steal their way into your mouth.

Amid all this bacterial bustle are your teeth, which come under attack when you eat. Bacteria, preying on sugars and starches, cling to teeth and form a sticky, colorless film called plaque. Plaque bacteria produce acids that can eat through enamel—the hard, white, mineral coating on the outside of your teeth. This creates a cavity.

Plaque can also irritate the *gingiva*, the gum tissue around the base of your teeth. When the gingiva becomes inflamed and bleeds easily, you have *gingivitis*.

Gingivitis can lead to a more serious condition called *periodontitis*. Both are forms of periodontal disease, which affects about three out of four adults over age 35. (Don't feel bad; about half of all high school students also have gingivitis.) With periodontitis, gums gradually withdraw from around your teeth. Tooth decay may develop on roots, which aren't protected by enamel. Also, ligaments and tooth sockets can become inflamed, potentially causing tooth loss.

Periodontal disease is treatable, especially if you and your dentist act early in the course of the disease. However, if unchecked, periodontal disease can precipitate or aggravate health problems elsewhere in the body. Indeed, recent studies suggest possible links to such problems as **heart disease**, **stroke**, **diabetes**, and **pneumonia**.

Special Dental Health Challenges for Older People

Many different factors put older people at greater risk for developing cavities, gum disease, and other dental health problems. Here are some of them:

- Aging fillings can lead to further tooth decay. (Your dentist may recommend replacing them.) Ill-fitting dentures can also impair oral health.

- As we age, we tend to take more medications. Many medications decrease saliva flow, which is the body's natural defense against cavities. (Decreased saliva flow also contributes to bad breath.)

- Some chronic diseases that are more common in older people can affect dental health. **Diabetes**, for example, can increase your risk for periodontal disease. If you have **arthritis** or other physical disabilities, pain and lack of flexibility may make it difficult for you to floss or brush your teeth. And people with **Alzheimer's disease** or other types of dementia may not remember to care for their teeth.

> ## WARNING SIGNS OF GUM DISEASE
>
> If you notice any of the following signs of gum disease, see your dentist:
>
> - gums that bleed when you brush your teeth
> - red, swollen, or tender gums
> - gums that have pulled away from the teeth
> - bad breath that doesn't go away
> - pus between your teeth and gums
> - loose teeth
> - a change in the way your teeth fit together when you bite
> - a change in the fit of partial dentures

- Fluoride, an element that helps prevent cavities, has been added to public water systems for decades. During your youth, however, you may not have been able to benefit from this public health measure. As a result, your teeth may have become riddled—and weakened—by cavities over the years. Even today you may not be receiving fluoride's benefits. You may not drink enough water. Or you may drink mostly fluoride-free bottled water or use water purifiers that remove fluoride.

- Growing up, you may not have been able to visit dentists regularly. As a result, your teeth and gums may not be as healthy today as they might have been. Your current dental care may also be inadequate. You may not have dental insurance and may see a dentist only when a problem develops.

- If you live alone, you may not eat as often or as nutritiously as you should. Eating a well-balanced diet helps keep teeth and gums healthy.

- You may lack transportation to a dentist's office, especially if you live in a nursing home. And your caregivers may not recognize that you need regular dental care.

Tips for Brushing and Caring for Gums

The biggest tip is no surprise and one you have been told your whole life: Brush your teeth at least twice a day, preferably after every meal, and remember to floss afterward.

More tips:

CAUTION

Avoid brushing your teeth too hard. It can wear down the tooth's root surface, making it more sensitive. To tell if you are brushing too hard, check the bristles on your brush. Do they point every which way but straight up? If so, then back off. Loosen your grip and use a softer-bristled toothbrush.

- Use a soft-bristled brush so you won't scratch your teeth's enamel.

- Place your brush at a 45-degree angle to your teeth, and use a short back-and-forth motion. Clean the inside of your teeth, tongue, and back teeth as well.

- Replace your brush when the bristles begin fraying—about every three to four months.

- To floss, ease the floss between your teeth. Form a "C" against the tooth's side, and gently rub the floss from the gum line to the top of the tooth. Remember to floss the back sides of your teeth and the teeth around a bridge (if you have one).

- Ask your dentist about prescription-strength fluoride rinses and treatments. Fluoride keeps teeth and gums healthy in all of us, no matter what our age.

- Don't avoid brushing if you have sensitive teeth. Ask your dentist about special toothpaste for sensitive teeth.

Special Brushing Tips If You Have Arthritis or a Disability

Don't let **arthritis**, **stroke**, or some other medical condition stop you from brushing and flossing your teeth. Your dentist can suggest adaptive devices, including extenders for toothbrush handles and specially designed floss holders. Or try the following "home remedies" recommended by the American Dental Association:

- Use a wide elastic band to attach the brush to your hand.

- Enlarge the brush handle with a sponge, small rubber ball, or bicycle handle grip. Also try winding an elastic bandage or adhesive tape around the handle.

- Lengthen the handle with a ruler, Popsicle stick, or tongue depressor.

- Tie the ends of the floss into a loop for easier handling.

- Use an electric toothbrush or commercial floss holder.

Do You Need a Dental Checkup?

Seeing a dentist regularly is critical for maintaining healthy teeth and gums. In addition to keeping cavities and periodontal disease in check, dentists are often the first to detect **oral cancer**, which occurs mainly in adults aged 45 and older.

How often you need to see a dentist depends on your health, medications (including over-the-counter drugs), and the condition of your teeth and gums. Some older people need to see their dentist every three months, while others may need only a yearly checkup.

Do you need a dental checkup? To find out, answer the questions at right.

Self-Test

Time to Call a Dentist?

Does your mouth feel unusually dry?
❑ Yes ❑ No

Do you have tooth or mouth pain?
❑ Yes ❑ No

Do you have lesions, sores, or lumps in your mouth?
❑ Yes ❑ No

Are your gums red, swollen, and painful?
❑ Yes ❑ No

Have you developed persistent bad breath?
❑ Yes ❑ No

Do you have a tooth that feels loose?
❑ Yes ❑ No

Has it been more than a year since you've seen a dentist?
❑ Yes ❑ No

If you answered "Yes" to any of these questions, call a dentist right away.

How to Choose a Dentist

Dental care should be very personalized. That kind of care begins with finding the right dentist. You want a dentist who is not only highly skilled, but who will also spend time answering your questions and putting you at ease.

Finding the right dentist means asking family, friends, or co-workers for recommendations. Your family physician or pharmacist may also give you leads.

Moving? Your current dentist may be able to recommend a dentist at your new location. Contact your local or state dental society. You can also use the American Dental Association's on-line member directory. The ADA Web site is www.ada.org.

Once you have a list of dentists, call or visit more than one before making a final decision. You will probably need to make appointments for these visits. Be aware that some dentists will charge you for an interview with them. So be sure to tell the office staff of your intent to interview the dentist when you schedule the appointment. Ask them up front what that fee will be.

Check out the office once you arrive. Is it clean, neat, and orderly? Is the location easy to reach from home or your job? Do the office hours fit your schedule? How friendly is the staff and the dentist? Do they encourage your questions and give you their attention? Are their explanations clear? Ask the dentist as many questions as you want, including the following:

- Do you explain techniques that will help me prevent dental health problems?

- What infection-control procedures do you use? The dentist should use "universal precautions" such as gloves, mask, and protective garb. Staff should routinely sterilize and disinfect instruments and the work area. In addition, the office should be in compliance with Occupational Safety and Health Administration (OSHA) regulations.

- Are my dental and medical histories recorded?

- What arrangements do you make for emergency dental care?

- Do you clearly explain treatment options and fees?

- Do you participate in my dental insurance program? What are my payment options?

- Is your office accessible to people with disabilities?

- If I have or develop a special health condition, do you have the interest, training, and experience to treat me?

Dental Bridges and Implants

Tooth loss happens. If it happens to you, don't hesitate to replace lost teeth. A full set of teeth helps you chew food better. It helps maintain a full smile. And it helps prevent a sagging face by providing support for lips and cheeks. Tooth gaps can cause your remaining teeth to change position, which can affect your bite and damage mouth tissues.

Dentists offer dental bridges and implants as options to filling the gap. A bridge attaches artificial teeth to adjacent natural teeth. Some bridges are permanent (fixed bridges); others are removable.

Dental implants are anchors that permanently hold replacement teeth. The most popular type of implants are metal screws surgically placed into the jawbones. Because implants attach so securely, they look and feel natural and offer excellent chewing ability. Candidates for implants must be in good health and have enough bone with which to secure the implant. Because bone heals slowly, treatment with implants often takes longer (four months to one year or more) than bridges or dentures.

Your dentist will help you decide which replacement option is best for you.

Taking Care of Dentures

About 32 million Americans wear full or partial dentures. Wearing dentures is nothing new. In one form or another they have been around for more than 2,000 years.

Dentures are durable, but not indestructible. So handle with care and follow these maintenance suggestions:

- Stand over a folded towel or a basin of water when handling dentures. Dropping dentures even a few inches can break a tooth or the denture base.

- When you remove your dentures at night, place them in a container of denture-cleaning solution or water. Dentures can warp if placed in hot water. If they become dried out, they may change shape and not fit properly.

- To clean, first rinse away loose food particles thoroughly. Brush your dentures to prevent staining and to keep your mouth healthy. Use a brush designed for dentures or a toothbrush with soft bristles. Use a denture cleaner rather than toothpaste. Some toothpastes may be too abrasive for dentures. Hand soap or mild dishwashing liquid are acceptable. Avoid using powdered household cleansers, which may be too abrasive.

- You can also use an ultrasonic cleaner. This type of cleaning should not, however, replace a thorough daily brushing.

- Don't try to adjust or repair dentures yourself. Improperly relined dentures can be bulky, causing increased pressure on the jaw and more rapid loss of jawbone.

- When not wearing your dentures, store them away from children and pets.

How to Banish Bad Breath

Some days you may wonder how a dragon got inside your mouth. Bad breath, or *halitosis*, has a long list of causes, including smoking, eating certain foods (such as garlic or onions), poor oral hygiene, gum disease, a dry mouth, medications, and medical disorders. People with a sinus infection, postnasal drip, or a respiratory-tract infection may also have bad breath.

How can you expel that dragon from your mouth? Watch what you eat and when. Also pay attention to when you don't eat: Infrequent eating can sometimes lead to unpleasant breath. If you smoke, stop. Your breath (not to mention your health) will benefit. And brush and floss regularly and in earnest, as if your social life depended on it. It may!

When to Seek Help

- If you have bad breath and your gums are puffy or bleeding, or you have tooth pain, sensitivity, or decay ▶ *Call your dentist now.*

- If you have bad breath and have a fever, sore throat, nasal discharge, or other symptoms unrelated to your teeth or gums ▶ *Call your physician now.*

Over-the-counter mouth rinses can offer temporary relief by masking the odor. But if you have a persistent or recurring case of bad breath, you should see your dentist. It's important to identify and treat the underlying cause of the odor.

Regular checkups will allow your dentist to detect any problems such as tooth decay, gum disease, a dry mouth, or other disorders that may be causing the halitosis. If you suffer from dry mouth, your dentist may prescribe an artificial saliva or suggest you suck on sugarless candy to keep the saliva flowing. Keeping your mouth moist and using a humidifier during dry winter months can also help. If you have postnasal drip, your dentist may recommend a moisturizing nasal spray.

At your regular checkup you should also receive a professional tooth cleaning from a dental hygienist. These cleanings are essential to reducing bad breath. The hygienist or your dentist may also recommend that you use a special antimicrobial mouth rinse at home.

Finally, your dentist may refer you to a doctor for evaluation and treatment of a medical disorder. Bad breath is associated with **diabetes**, gastrointestinal disturbance, and liver or kidney ailments.

Dental Specialties

Most of the more than 140,000 dentists in the United States practice general dentistry. They provide comprehensive care to a wide variety of people. Typically, you see your general dentist for regular checkups and cleanings and for minor, yet comprehensive, dental surgery. If a dental problem becomes too complex and needs specialized treatment, your dentist may refer you to a dental specialist. These specialists limit their practices to one of eight recognized dental specialties (p. 250).

Afraid of Going to the Dentist? Don't Be.

Many older people put off going to the dentist because they fear the visit will be painful. Often their anxiety is based on a bad experience they had years ago in a dentist's office.

Today, however, people need not fear the dentist's chair. New anesthetics and equipment can effectively block pain and minimize discomfort.

If you panic at the thought of going to the dentist, try these tips:

- Make the dental appointment at a time when you won't be rushed or preoccupied with other concerns—early in the morning, for example.

DENTISTS AND THEIR SPECIALTIES

Dentist	Specialty
Endodontist	Treatment of diseases and injuries of the dental pulp (commonly known as the nerve) and other dental tissues that affect the vitality of teeth
Oral and maxillofacial surgeons	Treatment of a broad range of diseases, injuries, and defects in the head, neck, face, jaws, and associated structures
Oral pathologist	Study and research of the causes, processes, and effects of diseases of the mouth; also provides diagnostic and consultative services
Orthodontist	Treatment of problems related to crooked teeth, missing teeth, and other abnormalities to establish normal function and appearance
Pediatric dentist	Treatment of dental problems in children, from birth through adolescence; may also treat people with certain disabilities beyond the age of adolescence
Periodontist	Treatment of diseases of the gums and bone supporting the teeth
Prosthodontist	Replacement of missing natural teeth with fixed or removable substitutes, such as dentures, bridges, and implants
Public health dentist	Prevention and control of dental disease and promotion of dental health through organized community efforts

Source: American Dental Association

- Ask a friend or family member to come with you so you'll feel more relaxed.

- Tell the dentist and his or her staff that you are feeling anxious. Let them know exactly what scares you, whether it's the sound of a drill or the fear of pain.

- Practice deep-breathing or other relaxation techniques while you are in the dental chair.

- Keep yourself distracted. Many dental offices offer their patients small radios or tape players with earphones. Some offices also have special glasses that allow you to watch videos during dental procedures.

Mouth Problems

EVEN if your teeth and gums are in tip-top shape, you can still experience annoying and usually minor mouth problems. Don't try to grin and bear these problems. Relief is just a dentist or doctor visit away.

Dry Mouth

Dry mouth, or *xerostomia*, is common, particularly among older people. The condition can make it hard to eat, swallow, taste, and speak. Dry mouth, which happens when salivary glands fail to work properly, can also contribute to tooth decay, poor digestion, and infection. It is usually a temporary condition.

Common causes of dry mouth include salivary gland infections, various diseases, and radiation therapy and chemotherapy. Dry mouth is also a side effect of more than 400 commonly used medicines, including drugs for **high blood pressure**, diuretics, antidepressants, antihistamines, and antireflux drugs.

Once, dry mouth was considered a normal part of aging. We now know that healthy older people produce as much saliva as younger adults. So if you think you have dry mouth, talk with your dentist or doctor. To relieve the dryness, drink extra water. Avoid sugary snacks, beverages with caffeine, tobacco, and alcohol—all of which increase dryness in the mouth. Sometimes, chewing sugarless gum, sucking on ice cubes, or rinsing with warm or salt water can stimulate saliva output. Your doctor or dentist may also prescribe an artificial saliva.

Mouth Pain and Infections

Most mouth pain involves tooth decay and inflamed gums. But sometimes the source of the pain may be a jagged tooth or badly fitting dentures. Cracks at the corners of your mouth can also result in mouth pain. Poorly fitting dentures or a vitamin deficiency can cause these cracks. Check with your dentist.

The tongue can also become sore. If your tongue is sore all over, you may have *glossitis*, an inflammation caused by infection, allergies, or poor nutrition. See a

When to Seek Help

- If an undiagnosed mouth sore persists for two weeks ▶ *Call your physician or dentist.*

- If you suspect medication may be causing mouth sores ▶ *Call your physician or dentist.*

doctor for treatment, and avoid hot, spicy foods, alcohol, and tobacco. These substances can irritate the tongue.

A white, splotchy tongue may be a sign of a condition known as *leukoplakia*. It causes white, usually wet, crusty patches to form on the tongue. The patches sometimes evolve into cancer. A velvety red patch in the mouth may indicate another condition known as *erythroplakia*. It is always considered precancerous and occurs most often in people 60 to 70 years of age. Both erythroplakia and leukoplakia are strongly associated with tobacco and alcohol use. These conditions are treatable but should receive care as soon as possible.

Occasionally you may develop creamy, yellow, slightly raised patches on the insides of your cheeks. If you rub them off when brushing your teeth or eating, raw and painful areas remain. This is called oral thrush, or *candidiasis*. The cause is a yeasty fungus, which is normally kept in check by the body. If your resistance is lowered or if you take certain antibiotics that destroy fungus-killing bacteria, this fungus may multiply out of control. You will require prescription treatment, usually antifungal lozenges or mouthwash.

If you find a lump in your mouth, it may be a benign tumor, a cyst, or (rarely) lichen planus, which is a white network of raised tissue. A lump can also be a sign of **oral cancer**. Don't try to determine what it is all by yourself. See a doctor.

Mouth Ulcers

Mouth ulcers, or sores, are common—and painful. Often looking like small, white craters, they break up the lining of the mouth and expose the sensitive tissue underneath. They can make eating and talking painful. If they can be easily seen, they can also cause embarrassment. The two most common mouth ulcers are cold sores and cankers.

Cold Sores

Cold sores are sometimes called "fever blisters" because they often erupt after an illness. Cold sores can show up anywhere on your body. However, they are most likely to appear on the outer, dry parts of the mouth, particularly your lips. The cause is usually the herpes simplex I virus, which cannot be cured or killed. The body keeps the virus in check most of the time, but when resistance drops because of stress, exhaustion, poor nutrition, food sensitivities, sunburn, fever, and so forth, the virus becomes active and you develop cold sores.

Cold sores are uncomfortable and at times unsightly, but they are not dangerous—provided the infection does not spread to your eyes, where it can cause blindness. In very rare cases, the herpes virus can infect the brain and other parts of the central nervous system. This can trigger meningitis and encephalitis, two life-threatening conditions. This complication is usually seen, however, only in adults with an immune deficiency disorder.

Cold sores usually last a week to 10 days. An antiviral agent may speed healing, however, if applied at the first sign of an outbreak. Applying ice to the sore or using an over-the-counter remedy that contains phenol can help relieve pain. To speed healing, try a water-based zinc ointment. Your doctor, dentist, or pharmacist can help you choose which medication is best for you. Using lip balm with a good sunscreen may help prevent future outbreaks.

Cold sores are highly contagious. Avoid kissing someone who has a cold sore; also, avoid using the same towels, toothpaste, razors, or utensils. Always wash your hands after touching a cold sore. And never rub your eyes or touch your genitals after touching your cold sore. You could develop corneal herpes or genital herpes.

Canker Sores

These small, shallow ulcers develop inside your mouth, on the moist tissue of the tongue, cheeks, or palate. Their cause is unknown, but they can become so painful that you do not want to eat.

People with a weakened immune system, a nutritional problem (especially deficiencies of vitamin B12, folic acid, or iron), and various gastrointestinal diseases appear to be at a higher risk for developing canker sores. Some research suggests that stress or skin injury may also contribute to their eruption in the mouth. And certain foods, especially citrus fruits, tomatoes, and some nuts, may make them worse in some people.

Canker sores are not contagious. To relieve the pain, try an over-the-counter medication that contains phenol. An antiseptic mouthwash or a mouth rinse consisting of warm water and salt will also help canker sores. Avoid eating hot, highly spiced foods or sharp, acidic foods until the sores have healed. If the pain persists or is severe, see your physician or dentist. He or she may prescribe an ointment or paste containing corticosteroids or tetracycline to lessen inflammation or a salve containing a local anesthetic.

Oral Cancer

ORAL cancer can strike people at any age but occurs most often in people over age 40. The incidence of the disease rises steadily with age, reaching a peak in people aged 65 to 74. For African Americans, the peak comes about a decade earlier. Oral cancer represents about 8 percent of all cancers. Men are twice as likely as women to develop this type of cancer.

Causes

Smoking and chewing tobacco are the main causes of oral cancer. People who smoke or chew tobacco regularly are 35 times more likely to get oral cancer than people who do neither. The risk to pipe and cigar smokers is as great as or greater than that to cigarette smokers. Inhaling snuff or drinking excessive amounts of

Symptoms

- A sore on the lip or in the mouth that does not heal
- A lump on the lip or in the mouth or throat
- A white or red patch on the gums, tongue, or lining of the mouth
- Unusual bleeding, pain, or numbness in the mouth
- A sore throat that does not go away, or a feeling that something is caught in the throat
- Difficulty or pain with chewing or swallowing
- Swelling of the jaw that causes dentures to fit poorly or become uncomfortable
- A change in the voice
- Pain in the ear that does not respond to treatment

When to Seek Help

- If you have any sores on the face, neck, or mouth that do not heal within two weeks

  ▶ *Call your physician or dentist.*

- If you have swellings, lumps, or bumps on the lips, gums, or other areas inside the mouth

  ▶ *Call your physician or dentist.*

- If you have white, red, or dark patches in the mouth

  ▶ *Call your physician or dentist.*

- If you have repeated bleeding in the mouth

  ▶ *Call your physician or dentist.*

- If you have numbness, loss of feeling, or pain in any area of the mouth

  ▶ *Call your physician or dentist.*

- If you have persistent hoarseness, soreness, or a feeling that something is lodged in your throat

  ▶ *Call your physician.*

alcohol also raises the risk. Some studies have shown that people with a history of leukoplakia (white patches in the mouth) or erythroplakia (red patches in the mouth) also have a greater chance of developing this type of cancer.

The disease usually affects tissue that is already irritated by jagged teeth, poor oral hygiene, ill-fitting dentures, and habitual chewing on the inside of the mouth. Iron deficiency is linked to tongue cancer in women, and excessive exposure to sunlight causes some types of lip cancer. Pipe smokers are especially prone to lip cancer.

Diagnosis and Treatment

A doctor will do a biopsy by taking a small tissue sample from your mouth. This tissue is then examined under a microscope. The doctor may also do X-rays or other imaging tests to identify tumors.

Small oral cancers respond equally well to surgery or radiation therapy. Radiation therapy can cause dry mouth. Laser surgery or cryosurgery (freezing cells with liquid nitrogen) can kill small tumors. Early detection is really important to avoid extensive surgery, which may result in facial disfigurement; reconstructive surgery may then be necessary. You may also need rehabilitation therapy to help you regain your ability to chew, swallow, and speak.

When oral cancer is found and treated early, the outlook is good. Three-fourths of cases are cured with early detection, and more than half the people with oral cancer survive for more than five years after treatment.

Prevention

- Don't smoke or chew tobacco.

- Drink alcohol only moderately, if at all.

- If you wear dentures, make sure they fit properly.

- Practice good oral hygiene.

- Use sunscreen to protect your lips.

- Eat fruits and vegetables high in vitamins A and E, which may be protective.

- If you have a precancerous abnormality, monitor it closely with your doctor.

Temporomandibular Disorders (TMD)

TEMPOROMANDIBULAR disorders are a group of often painful conditions that affect the jaw joint (also known as the *temporomandibular joint*, or *TMJ*) and the muscles that control chewing. The pain may happen suddenly, or it may develop slowly over a period of months or even years. About three-quarters of the people in the United States experience one or more symptoms of TMD at some time in their lives. Women are twice as likely as men to develop the disorder. Usually the problem goes away with little or no medical attention. But in about 5 percent to 10 percent of TMD cases, the pain persists and requires professional treatment.

Researchers have divided temporomandibular disorders into three main categories. *Myofascial pain* is the most common form of TMD. It involves discomfort or pain in the muscles that control the jaw, neck, and shoulders. *Internal derangement of the joint* refers to discomfort or pain caused by a dislocated jaw, a displaced jaw disk, or an injury to the lower jaw. *Degenerative joint disease* is pain caused by osteoarthritis or rheumatoid **arthritis** in the jaw joint. You can have more than one of these conditions at the same time.

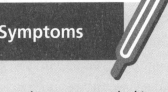

Symptoms

- Limited movement or locking of the jaw

- Persistent, radiating pain in the face, neck, or shoulders

- Painful clicking, popping, or grating sounds when opening your mouth or working the jaw

- A sudden, major change in the way the upper and lower teeth fit together

- Recurring **headaches**

> ## When to Seek Help
>
> - If you have a persistent jaw ache that does not respond to painkillers, heat, massage, or rest ▶ *Call your physician or dentist.*
>
> - If you have difficulty opening your mouth after an injury or blow to the face ▶ *Call your physician or dentist.*
>
> - If your jaw locks in certain positions ▶ *Call your physician or dentist.*

Causes

A heavy blow or other severe injury to the jaw can cause TMD. Joint diseases, such as **arthritis**, can also cause the disorder. Other causes of TMD are less clear. Some experts believe that stress, either emotional or physical, may cause or worsen TMD symptoms. People with TMD often clench or grind their teeth at night. This can tire the jaw muscles and lead to pain.

Recent studies have found no connection between a bad bite (*malocclusion*) and TMD. Nor is there any scientific proof linking TMD with gum chewing or jaw clicking. People with a jaw that pops or clicks most likely have a displaced jaw disk. But if the disk causes no pain and does not interfere with jaw movement, no treatment is needed.

Treatment

Because most cases of TMD are temporary, your best treatment is usually some simple self-care measures. To ease symptoms, apply moist heat to the face and eat soft foods. Also, avoid extreme jaw movements, such as wide yawning, gum chewing, and loud singing. Stress-reducing techniques such as biofeedback and yoga may also be helpful.

Your dentist or doctor may recommend short-term use of muscle-relaxing and anti-inflammatory drugs. You may also be given an oral appliance, also called a "splint" or "bite plate," to prevent teeth clenching or grinding.

In severe cases, you may need jaw surgery. Such surgery is irreversible and should be avoided when possible. Be sure you discuss its risk and benefits thoroughly with your physician. And be sure to get a second opinion from another qualified surgeon.

Prevention

- Avoid leaning or sleeping on your jaw. This practice is common among people who sleep on their stomachs. Try instead to sleep on your side or on your back.

- When your jaw hurts, talk as little as possible. Also, avoid gum and hard-to-chew foods, such as bagels.

- Avoid biting your nails and nibbling on pencils or other objects. This forces your jaw into an awkward position and may cause pain.

- Maintain good posture. Make sure your ear, shoulder, and hip are in a straight line while sitting and standing.

- Don't cradle a telephone receiver between your shoulder and jaw.

- If you feel jaw tension every morning, you may be grinding or clenching your teeth during the night. Talk to your dentist about wearing a bite guard.

- Rest your jaw from time to time. Keep your teeth apart, lips closed, and tongue on the roof of your mouth.

On Your Mind

Many people over the age of 50 can remember the severe stigma that used to be attached to **depression**, **alcoholism**, **anxiety**, and other mental health problems—and how that stigma often affected jobs, marriages, and life itself.

Today, most people do not dismiss mental illness as something that is "all in your head." Nor do they see having a mental illness as a moral failing. They may suffer from a mental illness themselves or know someone in their family who does (or did).

If you have a mental illness, you are not alone. Here are some eye-opening facts from a recent groundbreaking report by the U.S. Surgeon General:

- More than one in five Americans suffer from some form of mental illness.

- Half of Americans will suffer from a mental illness in their lifetime.

- Mental illness is second only to **coronary heart disease** as the leading cause of disability.

The report is more than statistics. In it the federal government recognizes the impact mental illness has on society, just as an earlier report from the Surgeon General acknowledged the impact that smoking has on our health.

This new report concludes that hope and treatment exist for nearly all mental disorders, including the most severe. The report's main recommendation is to seek help if you experience symptoms of mental illness.

Seeking help for mental illness does not come naturally to most people. According to the Surgeon General, a shocking two-thirds of people with mental illness never seek help. They suffer needlessly. Some people simply are unaware that they have a mental disorder; they don't hurt, exactly, or don't appear to have anything broken. They may not realize that effective treatment exists. Other people may be aware that they have a problem but do not seek help because they lack insurance that would cover mental illness.

Finally, let's not underestimate stigma. People still fear discrimination because of the stigma attached to mental illness. The Surgeon General's report reassures us that mental disorders are not character flaws, but legitimate illnesses. It also says that the "cruel and unfair stigma attached to mental illness" is "inexcusably outmoded." Such a stigma must no longer be tolerated.

Aging and Mental Health

MENTAL illness should not be confused with unhappiness. After experiencing life for 50 or more years, most of us understand that unhappiness, loss, frustrations, disappointments, and the "blues" are part of the deal. But sometimes unhappiness stays too long, changing to an enduring misery. It then refuses to move on. That's mental illness, in one form or another.

For some older people, the challenges of aging can contribute to **anxiety**, **depression**, and **grief**. Namely:

- The losses of life—whether through divorce, retirement, children gone from the nest, or the death of family members and dear friends—can play havoc with your emotions.

- You may be exhausted, sandwiched between ailing parents and family struggles.

- Retirement may have stopped you from doing what you enjoy, reduced contact with friends and colleagues, and caused financial stress.

- Possible physical problems—chronic illness, loss of hearing, diminishing eyesight—can drain your spirits.

- Certain medications can trigger **depression** and **anxiety**.

- You may not be able to do things—or remember—as well as you once could. And in a youth-oriented society, you may feel ashamed, powerless, and out of control because your possibilities seem to be dwindling.

These challenges are often offset, however, by the opportunities that come with aging to improve your mental health. This may be a time for caring for yourself, finally. You may now have the schedule, resources, focus, and determination that you did not have when you were younger. This can be your time to reflect on your life, celebrate, and put matters in order. Putting matters in order may include becoming devoted to the care of your body and mind.

Caring for Your Mental Health

A wide range of professional and lay resources are available to help people with mental health problems.

- Family doctors. Many mental health problems have a physical cause. Your doctor can review your medical history and medications for clues, provide basic counseling, prescribe medications, and, if necessary, refer you to other resources.

CAUTION

In some states, a person may use certain therapist titles without possessing specific credentials. Before being treated by mental health professionals, check their credentials through the state licensing boards for each profession.

- Clergy. In times of emotional stress, you may find comfort in turning to your faith. Many clergy members have formal training in counseling, and most are experienced in emotional issues and can refer you to other resources.

- Support groups. Most communities offer support groups for people suffering from **grief**, **depression**, and other mental health problems. Talk to your physician for referrals. Or call your local hospital. You can also call your local chapter of the National Mental Health Association or the National Alliance for the Mentally Ill.

- Psychologists, social workers, and counselors. These professionals are specially trained to help you deal with mental health issues.

- Psychiatrists. These are physicians who specialize in mental disorders. They counsel patients, prescribe medications, and order medical treatments. The special nature of **depression** and other mental illnesses in older people has led to a new medical specialty—geriatric psychiatry.

In the following pages you can read about alcoholism, drug abuse, **anxiety** and **anxiety disorders**, **depression**, and **grief** and loss. There are many other mental health problems, but these are among the most common. Knowing about these mental illnesses may spur you to seek professional help. You probably do not hesitate to call a doctor when your back aches, or a dentist when your tooth aches. Now, the hope is you'll do the same act of self-care by seeking help if and when your spirit aches.

Alcohol Abuse

ALCOHOL abuse causes more health problems in the United States than all illegal drugs combined. Some 14 million adults—1 in every 13—suffer drinking-related problems, and nearly 100,000 Americans die each year because of alcohol abuse. Heavy drinking has been linked to **coronary heart disease**, **high blood pressure**, **stroke**, kidney disease, impotence, certain types of **cancer**, liver failure, and a wide variety of crimes and social and domestic problems.

Most older problem drinkers are chronic abusers—people who have been heavy users of alcohol for many years. But some older people develop their drinking problem late in life. Often they drink to relieve the emotional pain of some situational factor, such as loneliness, the death of a loved one, retirement, or failing health. At first the drinking seems under control, but later it turns into a problem. In addition, alcohol has a bigger impact on your body—and your behavior—as you age. Even small amounts of alcohol can lead to big problems.

In older people, drinking problems often go undetected. That's because many of its consequences (blackouts, memory loss, fights with family members, and so on) are often mistaken for **Alzheimer's disease** or passed off as old-age "grumpiness." And many physicians, not wanting to embarrass their older patients, don't ask them about their drinking habits.

Symptoms

- A strong need, or compulsion, to drink

- Frequent inability to stop drinking once a person has begun

- Nausea, sweating, shakiness, **headaches**, and **anxiety** when alcohol use is stopped after a period of heavy drinking

- The need for increasing amounts of alcohol in order to get "high"

When to Seek Help

- If you have symptoms of alcoholism (opposite) and cannot stop drinking on your own

  ▶ *Call your nurse information service or physician.*

- If you tried to stop drinking and had symptoms of withdrawal (nausea, sweating, shakiness, **headaches**, and **anxiety**)

  ▶ *Call your nurse information service or physician.*

Causes

Alcoholism is a disease, not a character flaw. The causes are unclear, but there seems to be a blend of physical, psychological, environmental, and social factors involved. Heredity is a major factor. Your risk of becoming an alcoholic is four to five times greater if you had a parent who was an alcoholic.

Treatment

Abstinence is the goal of treatment. Treatment involves withdrawal and recovery. Withdrawal does not stop the craving for alcohol, and recovery may be marked with **anxiety** and **sleep problems**. Some people also experience uncontrollable shaking, spasms, panic, and the hallucinations of delirium tremens (DT).

Certain medications may be helpful. One (naltrexone) reduces the craving for alcohol. Another (disulfiram) interferes with alcohol metabolism so that drinking small amounts of alcohol causes nausea and vomiting. Antianxiety drugs and anti-depressants are also commonly prescribed.

Abstinence can be extremely difficult. Treatment can't begin until an alcoholic admits to having a problem, agrees to stop drinking, and then seeks help. This is why alcoholism has been called the most treatable untreated disease in America.

However, among alcoholics with otherwise good health, social support, and motivation, the chance of recovery is good. The recovery success rate for older people is particularly good because they tend to stay with treatment programs once they decide to seek help. Many alcoholics find invaluable support by attending such groups as Alcoholics Anonymous. The key is to find reliable support so you don't have to recover alone.

Self-Test

Do You Have an Alcohol Problem?

Have you ever felt you should cut down on your drinking?
❏ Yes ❏ No

Have people annoyed you by criticizing your drinking?
❏ Yes ❏ No

Have you ever felt bad or guilty about your drinking?
❏ Yes ❏ No

Have you ever had a drink first thing in the morning to steady your nerves or to get rid of a hangover?
❏ Yes ❏ No

One "yes" response suggests a possible alcohol problem. More than one "yes" response means it is highly likely that a problem exists. In either case, see your doctor to discuss your responses. He or she can help you determine whether you have a drinking problem and, if so, recommend the best course of action for you.

Even if you answered "no" to all of the questions, you should still seek professional help if you are encountering drinking-related problems with your job, relationships, health, or the law. The effects of alcohol abuse can be extremely serious—even fatal—both to you and to others.

Source: National Institute on Alcohol Abuse and Alcoholism

Prevention

- Don't underestimate the effects of alcohol.

- Don't drink to try to escape **anxiety** or **depression**.

- Avoid people and places that make drinking seem normal. Find new, nondrinking friends and activities.

- Ask for help from family and friends.

- Ask your doctor for advice about programs, foods, and vitamins that can aid in your recovery.

- Exercise regularly. Exercise releases chemicals in the brain that provide a natural "high" and reduce **anxiety**.

DRUG ABUSE: A HIDDEN PROBLEM

Drug abuse among older adults has been called an "invisible epidemic." The rate of misuse and abuse of prescription and other drugs is much higher for people aged 55 and older than it is for younger adults. But among older adults, these problems are much less likely to be detected and treated.

Drug abuse is using chemical substances often enough or in large enough doses to cause physical, mental, emotional, or social harm. Addiction means loss of control over drug use.

Older people often become drug abusers or addicts unknowingly. Aging can cause a slowing of metabolism and excretion rate. This may make it easier to overdose and eventually lose control over drug use.

Two to three million Americans are addicted to prescription drugs, and hospitals have as many emergencies from abuse of legal drugs as from illegal drugs. Prescription drug misuse and abuse is especially prevalent among older adults, largely because more drugs are prescribed to them.

As with alcohol abuse, the causes of drug abuse are unclear. Physical, psychological, environmental, and social factors are involved, and there seems to be a strong genetic factor in drug abuse. Most experts consider drug abuse a disease, not a character flaw. Tolerance to some drugs increases with use, so chronic abusers have to take more drugs to get an effect. For most addictive drugs, drug use continues partly because users fear the pain of withdrawal.

Treatment is withdrawal and recovery. Withdrawal can take days or even weeks. This time can be very difficult, painful, and even dangerous without professional help. Recovery is remaining drug-free for an extended period.

Like alcoholics, drug abusers may be "hard cases" because they deny they have a problem—even when their lives are in danger. Successful treatment programs create social support, boost self-esteem, and train abusers to avoid situations that can cause a slip. Medications, psychotherapy, social counseling, and self-help groups like Narcotics Anonymous (p. 348) all help abusers.

Anxiety and Anxiety Disorders

FEELING anxious can be good. It may spur you to take needed action. However, too much anxiety is hard on the body, mind, and soul. Indeed, when anxiety is not linked to a real threat and persists indefinitely, it is a clinical disorder.

Unfortunately, anxiety is too common among older people. Normal worries that accompany advancing age—such as fear of dying, of losing a loved one, of being alone, and of financial failure—sometimes develop into a persistent feeling of anxiety. You may feel frightened, distressed, and uneasy for no apparent reason. If not treated, these disorders can have a dramatic effect on your life, severely diminishing your quality of life.

If you suffer from an anxiety disorder, you are not alone. These debilitating illnesses are the most common mental illnesses in America. They affect more than 19 million people each year.

Symptoms

- Fast heartbeat or breathing rate
- Worry or fear that something bad will happen
- Trouble concentrating and irritability
- Muscle tension and aches, trembling
- Diarrhea
- Dry mouth
- Excessive sweating or cold or clammy hands
- Eating too much or too little
- **Sleep problems**
- Feeling dizzy or light-headed
- Loss of sex drive

When to Seek Help

- If you feel troubled, anxious, or out of control to the point that you cannot function ▶ *Call your nurse information service or physician.*

- If your anxiety seems irrational or more extreme than the situation dictates ▶ *Call your nurse information service or physician.*

- If low-level anxiety lasts for weeks, your symptoms get worse, or you have a new symptom ▶ *Call your nurse information service or physician.*

- If your symptoms suddenly become severe, or if you have weight loss and bulging eyes ▶ *Call your nurse information service or physician.*

Anxiety disorders are divided into five basic types:

- Generalized anxiety disorder. People with this disorder experience constant (lasting more than six months), exaggerated worrisome thoughts about everyday events and activities. They may also have physical symptoms, such as fatigue, trembling, muscle tension, **headaches**, or nausea.

- Phobias. Some people have a *specific phobia*. They have a constant and irrational fear of a particular thing, such as confining spaces, heights, blood, insects, flying, or snakes. This fear causes them to avoid the object or situation in a way that limits their lives unnecessarily. Other people have a *social phobia*, an overwhelming and disabling fear of social situations.

- Panic disorder. People with this disorder experience repeated episodes of sudden and extreme fear, usually for no clear reason. Each episode typically lasts a short while and may be accompanied by physical symptoms, such as chest pain, heart palpitations, shortness of breath, dizziness, and abdominal distress. A panic attack may sometimes be mistaken for a heart attack.

- Obsessive-compulsive disorder. People with this disorder have persistent, irrational thoughts, such as fear of germs. They may also develop compulsive behaviors, such as hand washing or checking the door to make sure it is locked, that seem impossible to stop or control.

- Post-traumatic stress disorder. This disorder is triggered by a traumatic event, such as war, rape, or a natural disaster. Its symptoms vary but often include nightmares, flashbacks, numbing of emotions, depression, anger, and irritability.

Causes

The stress of a particular event can trigger an anxiety disorder. Anxiety can also be a learned response to a past trauma or conflict. Research shows there is a physical side to anxiety; certain food sensitivities and chemical changes in the body—as well as withdrawal from alcohol, tobacco, and other drugs—can trigger panic attacks and anxiety. Finally, heredity appears to play a role. Studies of identical twins show that if one twin has an anxiety disorder, the other twin has a 50 percent chance of being similarly afflicted.

Diagnosis and Treatment

Some medical conditions, such as **thyroid problems**, **coronary heart disease**, and *hyper-* or *hypocalcemia* (too much or too little calcium) can produce symptoms similar to those of anxiety. For that reason, your doctor will first want to give you a thorough medical exam.

Once all medical conditions are ruled out, your primary care physician or a mental health professional will prescribe a treatment for the anxiety. That treatment may involve drugs, psychotherapy, stress reduction, biofeedback, or behavior modification. Some people also find benefit in acupuncture, massage, meditation, and yoga.

Treatments for anxiety disorders are extremely effective, so don't delay in getting hclp.

Prevention

- Exercise daily. It's one of the most effective therapies for anxiety.

- Avoid alcohol. Also, lower your intake of sugar, chocolate, and caffeine.

- Say no. This will reduce stress by making your schedule less hectic.

- Get enough rest and sleep.

- Plan enjoyable activities. Don't just hope you can "fit them in."

- Record your symptoms and share them with friends. Good friends may be able to help you identify exactly what is causing your anxiety.

- Get involved in social or volunteer groups. Being alone can make matters seem worse than they are.

- Remember the times when you were brave. You have conquered fears before, and you can do it again.

- Understand that asking for help is an act of courage.

Depression

EVERYONE gets the blues now and then. But being *chronically* depressed is not a normal part of growing old. It is a common problem, however. Major depression affects about 18 million Americans each year, with women twice as likely to be affected as men. Among people aged 65 and older, as many as 3 out of 100 suffer from major depression.

Depression in older people is often overlooked or misdiagnosed. Frequently, doctors and older people themselves dismiss symptoms of depression as part of growing old or as getting senile. Depression can also be tricky to recognize, especially if older people "put on a happy face" during doctor visits.

The good news is that people who are depressed can get better with the right treatment. According to the American Psychiatric Association, 80 percent to 90

Symptoms

- An "empty" feeling, ongoing sadness, and anxiety
- Tiredness, lack of energy
- Loss of interest or pleasure in everyday activities, including sex
- Sleep problems, including very early morning waking
- Problems with eating and weight (gain or loss)
- A lot of crying
- Aches and pains that just won't go away
- A hard time focusing, remembering, or making decisions
- Feeling that the future looks grim; feeling guilty, helpless, or worthless
- Being irritable
- Thoughts of death or suicide; a suicide attempt

When to Seek Help

- If you feel suicidal

▶ *Seek emergency care immediately.*

- If any of the symptoms of depression (p. 275) last for more than two weeks

▶ *Call your nurse information service or physician.*

percent of all cases can be treated effectively. "Talk" therapies, drugs, or other methods of treatment can ease the pain of this debilitating disease. No one needs to suffer in silence.

Causes

Depression has many causes. A particular life event can bring on a depressive reaction. People who suddenly find themselves struggling with a death in the family, for example, or a move to a new home may become deeply depressed.

Some illnesses have been linked to depression. These include **Parkinson's disease**, **stroke**, **diabetes**, and **thyroid problems**. Depression can also be a side effect of prescription drugs, especially those used to treat **arthritis**, heart problems, **high blood pressure**, and **cancer**.

Genetics, too, can play a role. Studies suggest depression runs in families. In one study, 27 percent of depressed children had close relatives who suffered from mood disorders.

And sometimes people become depressed for no clear reason.

Treatment

If you have any symptoms or concerns about depression, see your doctor. Don't think that you'll "snap out of it" or that you are too old to be helped. Nor should you think that getting help is a sign of emotional weakness. Depression is an illness, and fortunately it's one that can be treated successfully.

Your doctor will give you a complete exam to see if there are medical or drug-related reasons for your depression. He or she may feel comfortable treating your depression or may suggest that you talk to a mental health specialist. If your doctor does not take your concerns about depression seriously, you should seek a second opinion.

There are three main types of treatment for major depression: psychotherapy, medication, and electroconvulsive therapy. Sometimes the treatments are combined. Not everyone responds to a particular treatment in the same way. If your symptoms do not improve after several weeks, you and your doctor should reevaluate your treatment plan. But remember: A treatment that will work for you is out there. Even the most seriously depressed person can return to a happier and more fulfilling life.

Psychotherapy involves talking with a trained therapist. It can be very helpful in treating depression, especially in less severe cases. The therapy aims to teach you how to overcome negative attitudes and feelings that might have led to your depression. It also helps you improve your relationships with others in an effort to lessen feelings of despair.

Medications moderate or correct chemical imbalances in the brain that affect mood. They may also improve sleep, appetite, energy levels, and concentration. Individuals respond to each medication differently, and sometimes more than one medication is needed to treat depression. Some medications can take 6 to 12 weeks before showing any real signs of progress. They may need to be used for six months or more after symptoms disappear.

Electroconvulsive therapy (ECT) is most often recommended when drug treatments can't be tolerated or when very rapid improvement is necessary. ECT, which works quickly in most people, is given as a series of treatments over a few weeks. Improved techniques have made this therapy much safer than in past years, although temporary or permanent memory loss can occur. Anesthesia and muscle relaxants are given to people undergoing ECT to protect them from pain and physical harm.

HOW TO HELP SOMEONE WHO IS DEPRESSED

- Encourage the person to make an appointment with a doctor, or make the appointment yourself. Also, offer to accompany the person for support.

- Encourage the person to stick with the treatment plan and prescribed medications. Improvement may take several weeks. If no improvement occurs, encourage the person to seek a different treatment rather than giving up.

- Give emotional support by listening carefully and offering hope.

- Invite the person to join you in activities that you know he or she used to enjoy. Keep in mind, though, that expecting too much too soon may lead to feelings of failure.

- Don't accuse the person of faking illness or expect them to "snap out of it."

- Take comments about suicide seriously, and seek professional advice.

Source: National Institute of Mental Health

Prevention

Some forms of depression—those triggered by chemical malfunctioning in the brain—may not be preventable. But you may be able to prevent or ease many other forms of depression with good health habits, proper diet, exercise, vacations, not overworking, and protecting the time you set aside for activities you enjoy.

Here are some other practical steps you can take to overcome mild depression:

- To prepare for major changes in life—retirement or the death of family or friends—maintain friendships. Friends can help ease the loneliness of loss.

- Develop interests or hobbies to keep the mind and body active.

- Substitute positive thoughts for negative ones. And associate with friendly, positive people.

- Take a class and get involved at a senior center or your place of worship. Try to focus your attention away from yourself. Perhaps try something new and challenging.

- Follow your doctor's directions on using medicines. Doing so will help lower the risk of developing a drug-induced depression.

- Be physically fit and eat a balanced diet. This can help you avoid illnesses that can bring on disability or depression. Also, regularly do things that make you relax. Listen to soft music, read good books, and take warm baths.

LIGHTEN UP: SEASONAL AFFECTIVE DISORDER

Seasonal affective disorder, called *SAD*, is a type of depression that strikes only during the darkest half of the year. It starts in the fall, when days become shorter, and ends in the spring, when days become longer. In addition to depression, symptoms include energy loss, increased anxiety, oversleeping, and overeating.

The cause of SAD is not known, but scientists suspect it is linked to sunlight. Research suggests that decreased sunlight can affect our sleep cycle and brain chemicals, causing depression. This is borne out by studies comparing the incidence of SAD with where people live. SAD has been found to be more common in northern latitudes because the winter day gets shorter as you go farther north. In Florida, for example, less than 1 percent of the general population has SAD, while in Alaska as many as 10 percent of people may suffer from winter depression.

Several studies suggest that light therapy, which involves daily exposure to bright artificial light, may be an effective treatment for SAD. Sitting under a light box for as little as 30 minutes a day results in significant improvement in 60 percent to 80 percent of SAD patients. Light therapy is very safe, although people with certain medical conditions or who are taking certain medications should avoid it. Talk to your doctor before trying this therapy.

Here are other, self-help suggestions for SAD:

- Take a walk at lunch, when the sun is high. Be outdoors as often as you can. (But remember to wear sunscreen!)

- Exercise regularly.

- Take winter vacations in places with long days.

- Increase the natural light in your home by trimming low-lying branches near the house and hedges around the windows.

- Paint your walls with lighter colors.

- If all else fails, move to a sunnier climate.

Grief and Loss

GRIEF is an emotion that almost all older people know. You probably have lost someone close—a parent, spouse, or sibling, perhaps—and you know the deep pain of such a loss. You may also know the grief that comes with divorce, miscarriage or stillbirth, the end of a friendship or serious relationship, a disabling illness or accident, or the loss of a pet.

Unfortunately, grieving is a part of living. It is normal to grieve after a loss. Grief, particularly after the death of a loved one, often occurs in stages. The first is a mixture of shock, numbness, and denial. You cannot or will not believe that the death has occurred. You may feel drained, lonely, hopeless, or as if you are in a trance. You neglect yourself because you are unable to decide or take action. This neglect can stress the immune system, or may turn to **depression** or another illness. It can also lead to an accident.

Symptoms

- **Depression** and fatigue
- Sudden shifts in emotions
- Feeling helpless, lost, and out of control
- **Sleep problems**
- Physical pain or discomfort; vague feelings of illness
- Overeating or loss of appetite
- Trouble focusing or making decisions
- Self-destructive behavior, such as reckless driving and abuse of alcohol and drugs
- Hallucinations

When to Seek Help

- If you feel suicidal ▶ *Seek emergency care immediately.*

- If symptoms of grief and loss (opposite) last longer than two weeks ▶ *Call your nurse information service or physician.*

The later phases of grief include equally intense feelings, such as the following:

- Anger at the unfairness of the death or even at the deceased for leaving you. Your anger may drive others away, heightening your loneliness.

- Fear of loneliness, of your own death, or that other loved ones may also die.

- Guilt that you survived and the deceased did not. Or you may have guilt about past wrongs involving the deceased that you wish you could have made right.

Treatment

Treatment is often passive. That is, let grief happen. Allow yourself, experts advise, to feel numb, sad, angry—whatever the emotion is. Let it out. Too often, people want to do whatever it takes to avoid grief. Often that avoidance backfires, and more emotional problems develop. Don't go around grief, say the experts; go through it.

Gradually, at your own pace but usually within two years, acceptance sets in. You adjust to the loss and begin to make positive plans for the future. This process can involve periods of pain and heartache (particularly during holidays and anniversaries), but eventually grief's grip over you will release.

Family and friends can often provide the support needed for full recovery. But you may also need help from social workers, doctors, grief support groups, and clergy. Mental health professionals can provide the psychotherapy and counseling needed for recovery. Psychiatrists may be necessary when **depression** and perhaps suicidal thoughts seem to block any chance of recovery.

At-Home Care

Grieving is personal. Everyone handles it his or her own way. The following suggestions, however, may provide some help:

- Share your grief with friends. The more friends the better; you don't want to "wear out" one friend with all your grief. Let several give you their support.

- Find a support group. Ask your doctor, clergy, or a mental health professional for a referral.

- Put off major decisions while you are grieving. You do not need to decide about moving or financial matters just now.

- Whether you feel like it or not, eat healthful foods. Eat with other people as often as you can. It's a great way to socialize and make sure you are eating a balanced meal.

- Try to get as much sleep as possible.

- Get some form of regular exercise.

- Go to or get back to work, or volunteer. It will take your mind off your troubles.

- Develop a green thumb. Plants and fresh flowers in the house help you think of life. Pets do, too.

- Dress in bright, cheerful colors.

- Don't stay in bed in the mornings. It's okay once in a while, but try to get up and out of the house at least once a day.

- If someone you love is dying, don't leave important things unsaid. Work to resolve as much as you can before the death.

HOW TO HELP A FRIEND WHO IS GRIEVING

- Support the friend with acts of comfort.

- Be a sympathetic and patient listener.

- If you don't know what to say, ask your friend how you can help.

- Avoid judging how the friend is grieving. Each of us grieves in a different way.

- Help with practical matters. Offer to shop for food, clean the house, or mow the lawn.

- Share activities with your friend.

- Avoid saying, "I know how you feel." Grief is very personal.

- If a friend is grieving the death of a loved one, don't assume it was for the best, no matter how old or ill the deceased was. Do talk about the deceased. Memories can be of great solace to the bereaved.

- Don't say, "It is God's will."

Mental Fitness

MENTAL fitness is like physical fitness. Just as you do certain activities (walk, garden, swim, bike) to keep the body in shape, you also can do certain activities to keep your mind and mental outlook in tip-top form.

In other words, the adage we follow to achieve physical fitness also applies to mental fitness: "Use it or lose it!"

You Must Remember This

Growing older does not mean automatically losing your ability to think, reason, and remember. In fact, one interesting study compared memories of a group of 18- to 34-year-olds to memories of 57- to 83-year-olds. Researchers found that long-term memory—the kind that holds the overall store of information and experiences accumulated over a lifetime—was better in the older group than in the younger group!

That said, most people find that their memory slows down a bit as they age. Short-term memory ("Where did I put my glasses?") may take longer to work, and recollections of the past few days may be a bit fuzzy. This may be age-related. More often, however, the memory loss is related to stress, **depression**, medications, poor nutrition, changes related to retirement, or **grief**.

Keep in mind that forgetfulness is different from dementia, which is a serious decline in memory. To put it simply, forgetfulness is going to a wedding and forgetting the names of

Did You Know?

Eating foods rich in antioxidants (fruits and vegetables) may help prevent the natural decline in brain function that comes with growing older. Researchers have found that antioxidants protect against declines in nerve cell communications, which are important for memory performance.

some of the people there. Dementia is going to a wedding and forgetting you were even there. **Alzheimer's disease** and **stroke** are responsible for most cases of dementia.

Active Body, Active Brain

Exercise is one of the keys to keeping your mind sharp as you age. It helps preserve the blood supply to the brain. As a result, regular exercise can help you maintain quick reaction times and improve your thinking power. Numerous studies have shown this to be true.

One study from the University of Illinois found that previously sedentary people over age 60 who walked rapidly for at least 45 minutes three days a week significantly improved their mental processing abilities. The study's volunteers started by walking 15 minutes three times a week at a modest 17.7 minutes per mile. They then gradually worked up to walking 16-minute miles for 45 to 60 minutes three times a week.

This exercise regimen was enough to significantly increase blood flow—and thus oxygen—to the frontal regions of the brain. The increased oxygen caused the volunteers to have faster reaction times when completing a variety of mental tasks on a computer. They were found to be better able to ignore distractions—the same kind of mental skill needed when driving a car and doing many other daily tasks.

In another study, researchers tested the aerobic fitness levels of 132 volunteers between the ages of 24 and 76. They then gave them several mental tests. Although the younger volunteers completed the mental tasks more quickly, the more fit the older volunteers were, the faster their performances. Furthermore, the greater the age of the volunteer, the greater impact his or her fitness level had on performance.

Use It or Lose It

Here are suggestions for keeping your memory sharp:

- Do crossword puzzles and card games that require memory skills.

- Build routines into your day. Routines help you remember more.

- Use lists, which helps memory by keeping the mind free of clutter.

- Make associations, especially visual connections, between what you are trying to learn and what you know. Experts say the more ridiculous the association, the better the chances of remembering.

- Practice names. When you meet a new person, try to use the name right away: "Nice to meet you, Hank." Focusing and repetition are important to memory.

- Memorize something every day, be it a joke, poem, Scripture, or quotation.

- Learn a new language.

- When you forget, don't panic. Don't give up or try to rush recall. Tell yourself that it will come to you later, and it probably will.

- Have your doctor evaluate your medications. He or she may be able to make adjustments to improve your memory. Your doctor can also evaluate you for physical disorders, such as hypothyroidism, or mental disorders, such as **depression**, that can affect memory.

Medication Matters

Drugs have helped people live longer. In fact, you may owe your life to new and improved medications and vaccines.

But drugs have their downside, too. This is true especially for older people, who often take many different drugs prescribed by many different doctors for many different ailments. One survey reported that the average number of prescription drugs taken by residents in a senior citizen urban dwelling was 4.5 per person. They also took 3.4 nonprescription drugs for a total of 7.9 medications per day. It is estimated that people over age 65 buy 30 percent of all prescription drugs and 40 percent of all over-the-counter drugs. Keeping them straight can be a challenge.

Even when all these medications don't produce a bad mix, they are known to affect older people differently from younger people. As you age, you lose water and muscle tissue and gain fat. This can make a difference in how long a drug stays in your body and how much of it your body absorbs. Also, the kidneys and liver, which break down and remove drugs from the body, may not work as well as they used to.

Even though drugs are commonplace, don't underestimate their power and their risks to you. Many people do, which is why we have statistics such as these:

- About a quarter of all nursing home admissions are due, at least in part, to the inability to take medication correctly.

- One report stated that 51 percent of deaths from drug reactions involve people aged 60 and older. Also, some 200,000 older Americans are hospitalized each year because of adverse reactions to drugs.

- A person at age 65 is twice as likely to have unwanted side effects from medicines as someone at age 35; an 80-year-old is four times as likely to have undesired side effects.

Make sure you and your family learn about the drugs you take. The following tips can help you avoid risks and get the best results from your medicines.

Dos and Don'ts for Medication Safety

- DO take medicine in the exact amount and on the same schedule prescribed by your doctor.

- DO always ask your doctor about the right way to take any medicine before you start to use it.

- DO always tell your doctor about past problems you have had with drugs, such as rashes, **indigestion**, dizziness, or loss of appetite.

- DO keep a daily record of all the drugs you take. Include prescription and over-the-counter (OTC) drugs. Note the name of each drug, the doctor who prescribed it, the amount you take, and the times of day you take it. Keep a copy in your medicine cabinet and one in your wallet or pocketbook.

- DO review your drug record with the doctor at every visit and whenever your doctor prescribes new medicine. Your doctor often gets new information about drugs that might be important to you.

- DO make sure you can read and understand the drug name and the directions on the container. If the label is hard to read, ask your pharmacist to use large type.

- DO check the expiration dates on your medicine bottles. Throw the medicine away if it has passed this date.

- DO call your doctor right away if you have any problems with your medicines.

GET TO KNOW YOUR PHARMACIST

You should take every medication seriously, whether it was prescribed by a doctor or bought directly off the shelf at a drugstore. To help you do this in a personal way, get to know a pharmacist.

Find a pharmacist, preferably local, who seems competent and has the time to talk with you. That might mean finding an independent drugstore rather than one of the chains that specialize in volume rather than personal service.

Once you find the right pharmacist for you, fill all your prescriptions at that pharmacy. That way your pharmacist will have a computerized record of all your medication (including OTC drugs) on file and can alert you to any problems.

There are also some things you should remember not to do:

- DO NOT stop taking a prescription drug unless your doctor says it's okay—even if you are feeling better. If you are worried that the drug might be doing more harm than good, talk with your doctor. He or she may be able to change your medicine to another one that will work just as well.

- DO NOT take more or less than the prescribed amount of any drug.

- DO NOT mix alcohol and medicine unless your doctor says it's okay. Some drugs may not work well or may make you sick if taken with alcohol.

- DO NOT take drugs prescribed for another person or give yours to someone else.

Source: National Institute on Aging

Questions to Ask Your Doctor

Before leaving the doctor's office, ask these questions about medications:

- What is the name of the drug and what will it do?

- How often should I take it?

- How long should I take it?

- When should I take it? As needed? Before, with, after, or between meals? At bedtime?

- If I forget to take it, what should I do?

- What side effects might I expect? Should I report them?

- Are there other drugs or foods that might interact with this drug?

- Is there any material about this drug that I can take with me?

- If I don't take this drug, is there anything else that would work as well?

How to Use Over-the-Counter Medications

Headaches, **indigestion**, diarrhea, **colds**, and **flu**. You can find relief from these common ailments with over-the-counter medications. OTC medications include a variety of products, such as vitamins and minerals, laxatives, cold medicines, and antacids. Herbal medicines also fall into the OTC category.

Remember: A drug is still a drug, which means OTC medications have the same safety issues as prescription drugs. Follow these guidelines to ensure that you use OTC drugs safely and effectively.

- Talk to your doctor before taking an OTC medication. Taking this protective step is especially important for older people and people with chronic illnesses. Be sure to tell your doctor about any other OTC medications, including herbal ones, you are currently taking.

- Read product labels and follow instructions carefully.

- If you develop a rash or other allergic reaction while taking an OTC medication, stop taking it and call your doctor immediately.

Drug Reaction or Symptom?

Sometimes, what appear to be symptoms of an illness are really signs of an adverse reaction to a medication. If you experience any of the symptoms below soon after starting on a new medication, check with your doctor. You may not be ill, just in need of an adjustment in your medications.

- Diarrhea
- Vomiting
- Difficulty breathing
- Appetite loss
- Muscular weakness (which may cause a fall)
- Skin rashes and other allergic reactions
- Drowsiness, confusion, or memory loss
- Depression or sadness
- Difficulty sleeping

Safety and Dietary Supplements

About half of the adults in the United States use dietary supplements. Together, we spend nearly $7 billion a year on them. Some of these supplements are helpful in treating a variety of conditions and have received FDA approval. But many are not helpful—or at least their claims have yet to be proven. And some can be downright dangerous if misused or taken inappropriately.

FOODS THAT CAN INTERFERE WITH DRUGS

Food	Don't Mix with	What Can Happen	Recommendation
Alcohol	Certain antibiotics, pain relievers (acetaminophen), sleeping pills, and tranquilizers	Rapid pulse, low blood pressure, vomiting, confused thinking (antibiotics); possible liver damage, stomach bleeding (pain relievers); dizziness, severe drowsiness (sleeping pills, tranquilizers)	If you drink alcohol, consult your physician before taking pain relievers. Don't combine antibiotics, sleeping pills, or tranquilizers with alcohol.
Broccoli, cabbage, soybeans, and other Vitamin K-rich foods	Certain anticoagulants	Reduces effect of anticoagulant.	Check with your physician.
Dairy products	Certain antibiotics and some thyroid replacement drugs	Antibiotic may not work as well.	Wait 2 hours after eating dairy foods to take medication.
Grapefruit juice	Calcium channel-blockers (for **high blood pressure**) and cyclosporine (for rheumatoid **arthritis**, psoriasis, and other conditions)	Light-headedness, **headache**; increase of drug in blood	Don't take these drugs with grapefruit juice.
Liver, aged cheese, salted fish, red wine, and other tyramine-rich foods	Certain antidepressants (MAO inhibitors)	Rise in blood pressure, dizziness, nausea, bleeding	Don't mix these foods with these drugs.

The 1994 Dietary Supplement Health and Education Act (DSHEA) set up a new framework for FDA regulation of dietary supplements. It also created an office in the National Institutes of Health to coordinate research on these supplements. In passing DSHEA, Congress recognized 1) that many people believe dietary supplements offer health benefits; and 2) consumers want a greater opportunity to determine whether supplements are safe and effective.

That said, the FDA is limited in regulating dietary supplements. FDA's requirement for premarket review of dietary supplements is less than that of drugs and many additives used in conventional foods. This means that manufacturers and you, the consumer, also have a responsibility for checking the safety of dietary supplements and determining the truthfulness of any health claims on their labels.

So, be cautious about supplements. Always check with your doctor before taking them. And be on the lookout for fraudulent products. Here are some possible indicators of fraud, according to the National Council Against Health Fraud:

- Claims that the product is a secret cure. Such claims often include such words as "breakthrough," "magical," and "miracle cure." If the product really was so miraculous, you can be sure that the media would not keep it a secret.

- Claims that the product can "detoxify," "purify," or "energize." Such terms are vague and hard to measure, which makes it easier for the manufacturer to make unsubstantiated claims.

- Claims that a product can cure a number of wide-ranging diseases. No product can do that.

- Claims that a product is backed by scientific studies when no list of references is provided. Or if there is a list, an examination of the studies may show that some of the references are untraceable and others irrelevant or poorly designed.

- Claims that a supplement has only benefits with no side effects.

- Accusations that the government, medical profession, and drug companies are suppressing information about a treatment.

How to Take Antibiotics Effectively

Antibiotics are prescription drugs that kill bacteria. This large class of drugs has no effect on viruses and will not cure **colds**, **flu**, or any other viral illnesses.

Antibiotics have been a huge advance in medicine because they have helped control many infectious diseases. They have saved millions of lives. But as with any drug, antibiotics have their adverse effects. They can cause nausea, diarrhea, and allergic reactions. They can kill most bacteria in your body, including those that are helpful. And bacteria can become resistant to antibiotics when the drugs are prescribed too frequently or when only part of the prescription is taken.

So, when taking antibiotics, follow these directions:

- Take the whole dose for as many days as prescribed. Do this even if you feel better in a few days. Antibiotics kill off bacteria quickly, but if you stop taking them too soon, the stronger bacteria will survive and flourish. If you experience severe side effects, call your doctor.

- Make sure you understand all instructions about taking the medication. The instructions should be printed on the label, but also check with your doctor or pharmacist.

- Store antibiotics in a cool, dry place. They will usually last about a year. Liquid antibiotics are always dated. Check to see if they need refrigeration.

- Never share antibiotics. If they are prescribed for you, don't give them to a friend, who may develop serious side effects.

- If you have antibiotics prescribed for a particular illness, don't take them for another illness without your doctor's approval.

Storing and Caring for Your Medications

Heat and humidity are enemies of your medications. Store all medications in a cool, dry place, such as a closet shelf. Use a high shelf or a lock to keep them away from children. Don't store medications in the bathroom, where heat and humidity can get high.

Keep medications in their original containers. That way, you will avoid any confusion about what you are taking. Never put them near a dangerous substance, such as a cleaning product. You might take the substance by mistake.

Don't store medications in your car; temperatures inside your car can be as much as 50 degrees higher than outside. If you must transport medications in your car, keep them in an insulated container and out of direct sunlight.

Managing Your Medications

Here are tips for helping your medicines work as safely and effectively as possible:

- Keep a record of all current medicines, including name, dose, time, and other instructions for taking. Write down problems you may experience while taking the medicines. Give a copy of this list to every doctor and alternative health practitioner you see. Be sure to talk to your doctor or pharmacist about these problems.

- Always take your medicine in good light. Read labels carefully before taking doses. Carefully read OTC medicine labels for ingredients, proper uses, directions, warnings, precautions, and expiration dates.

- Ask your doctor or pharmacist before crushing or splitting tablets; some should only be swallowed whole.

- Never stop taking medicine the doctor has told you to finish just because your symptoms disappear.

- Ask your doctor periodically to reevaluate long-term treatments.

- Discard outdated medicine.

- Never take someone else's medicine.

- Tell each of your health professionals if you are allergic to drugs or foods, have **diabetes** or kidney or liver disease, follow a special diet or take dietary supplements, use alcohol or tobacco, or take other prescription or OTC medicines regularly. Show the doctors your medication containers with their labels.

- Don't buy a medication if the packaging is broken or looks as if it has been tampered with.

Develop a Medication Routine

Studies have shown that 40 percent to 75 percent of older people do not take their medications at the right time or in the right amount. To make sure you take your medications correctly, follow these suggestions:

- If you have **arthritis** or other disability, ask the pharmacist for an oversize, easy-to-open bottle.

- For easier reading, ask the pharmacist for large-type labels. If such labels are not available, use a magnifying glass and read medication labels in a well-lit room.

- Devise a system to remember medications. Make sure it's a system that fits your daily schedule. Use meals or bedtimes as cues for remembering. Set a timer or programmable beeper to remind you. Or ask a friend to give you a call at prearranged times. Make your own charts and calendars. Purchase weekly pillboxes, or use an egg carton or cupcake pan as a medication holder.

- Don't keep containers of pills on your bedside table unless it is absolutely necessary. It is too easy to grab the wrong container in the middle of the night or early in the morning, when you are still groggy.

- Don't leave similar-looking drug containers grouped together. If necessary, ask your pharmacist to change the packaging of a drug.

CAUTION

WARNING: NOT IN FRONT OF THE KIDS

Here's a startling statistic: Over one-third of childhood poisonings occur in a grandparent's home.

What can you do to make sure your grandchild is not one of those statistics? To begin with, don't take medications in front of small children. They like to mimic and often are not hesitant about putting something into their mouths that looks like candy.

Keep medication out of a child's reach. And women, if you keep your medications in your purse, be sure to keep your purse out of their reach, too.

By the way, those child-resistant caps do not always work. About 20 percent of accidental poisonings with children involve properly secured child-resistant caps.

- Try to do your own research on each drug you take. Check the library or go on-line to a reputable Web site.

Emergencies and First Aid

The first few minutes after an injury or medical crisis are often the most crucial. It's important to stay calm, evaluate the situation, then act. That action may mean calling the paramedics, applying pressure to stop bleeding, making a splint to stabilize a **broken bone**, or performing cardiopulmonary resuscitation (CPR). Never perform a medical procedure, however, if you are unsure how to do it.

Learn what to do *before* a medical emergency happens. Being prepared can help you take quick action, which can save a life. Here are some steps you should take to prepare yourself and your family for an emergency:

- Keep a list of emergency rescue numbers next to the telephone and in your pocket, wallet, or purse. In most communities, 911 is the number to call for all emergencies.

- Find out the location of, and the fastest route to, the emergency department nearest you for life-threatening situations. If there is more than one nearby, ask your doctor which one he or she recommends of those listed with your health care organization.

- Take a first-aid class. Learn CPR and other emergency care techniques. Call your local chapter of the American Heart Association or American Red Cross for information on classes.

- Keep a well-stocked first-aid kit in your home and in each of your family's cars.

- Make a list of all the medications you take and their dosages. Also list any medical conditions you have and/or any surgeries you have had. Carry this list with you and put copies in each of your first-aid kits. Make sure there is a list for each member of your family.

- Make a list of any allergies you have, especially drug allergies or those that result in severe reactions. Carry an EpiPen® or other device to treat anaphylactic shock if you have a history of severe allergic reactions.

- If you have a medical condition that requires special treatment in a medical emergency, be sure to wear a medical alert tag. Ask your doctor how to get one of these lifesaving tags.

WHAT TO DO IN AN EMERGENCY

1. Keep calm.

2. Quickly survey the scene for hazards (such as live electrical wires). Do not move the person unless absolutely necessary if you suspect a head, neck, or back injury.

3. Call 911 or your local emergency number, or send someone else to do so.

4. Do the ABCs of CPR (below).

5. Control bleeding (p. 304-305).

6. Prevent shock (p. 317).

7. Try to determine as much as you can about what caused the emergency. Pass this information on to the paramedics when they arrive.

The ABCs of CPR (Cardiopulmonary Resuscitation)

Cardiopulmonary resuscitation (CPR) is emergency treatment for someone who is not breathing and has no heartbeat. It opens the airway, reestablishes breathing, and gets blood circulating again. It can, quite literally, save lives.

At the scene of an emergency, the person who has the most experience and training in CPR should be the one to perform the procedure.

The steps of CPR are described here. These are intended only as a review; they are *not* a substitute for taking a detailed, hands-on CPR course. Every adult should learn CPR. It's never too late to get the training.

WARNING: Always call 911 before starting CPR. Also, never perform CPR unless a person's breathing and circulation (pulse) have stopped.

Step 1: A = Airway

Gently open the airway by tilting the person's head back. *Caution:* If you suspect a head, neck, or back injury, lift only the chin.

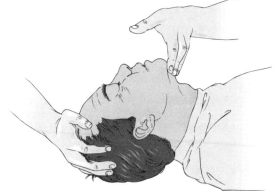

Step 2: B = Breathing

Look, listen, and feel for signs of breathing. If there are no signs of breathing, pinch the person's nose and give two strong breaths into his or her mouth. Check that the rib cage rises with each breath. If this does not happen, repeat Step 1.

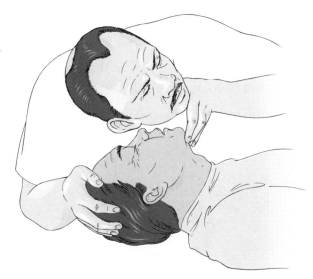

Step 3: C = Circulation

Check for a pulse at the neck.* To do this, place two fingers in the depression on the side of the neck beneath the jaw. If there is a pulse, give the person mouth-to-mouth breathing until breathing returns.

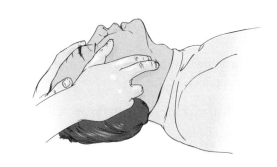

continued on next page

*NOTE: The American Heart Association (AHA) is in the process of revising this step in their CPR procedure. For more information, contact the AHA (p. 345).

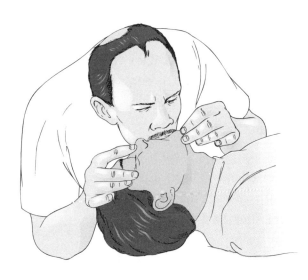

If there is no pulse, lay the person flat on his or her back and start chest compression:

- Kneel beside the person. Find the base of the person's *sternum*—the point where all the ribs come together in the center of the chest.

- Put two fingers on that point. Put the heel of your palm beside those two fingers.

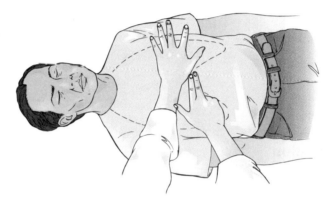

- Place the heel of your other palm on top of the first. Your fingers should not touch the chest.

- With arms straight, lean forward until your shoulders are above the person's breastbone.

- Press the breastbone downward about two inches.

- With your hands in place, lean back and let the breastbone rise to its original position.

- Give 15 compressions at the count of "one and two and three and…."

- Give two strong breaths into the person's mouth.

- Continue giving 15 compressions followed by two breaths until pulse returns. (Check the pulse at the neck after the first minute and then after every three minutes.)

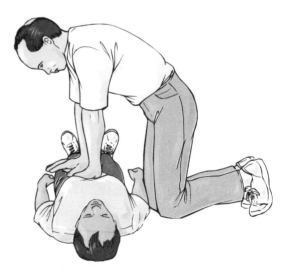

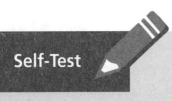

Self-Test

Should You Call an Ambulance or Drive to the Emergency Room?

Is the victim's condition life-threatening?

❑ Yes ❑ No

Could the victim's condition worsen and become life-threatening on the way to the hospital?

❑ Yes ❑ No

Could moving the victim require the skills or equipment of paramedics or emergency medical technicians?

❑ Yes ❑ No

Would distance or traffic conditions cause a delay in getting the victim to the hospital?

❑ Yes ❑ No

If the answer to any of these questions is "yes," or if you are unsure, it's best to call an ambulance.

Source: American College of Emergency Physicians

YOUR FIRST-AID KIT

One of the best ways to prepare for emergencies is to have a home first-aid kit. It's also a good idea to stow a first-aid kit in each of your family's cars. Kits should contain the following:

Information

- Emergency phone numbers, including numbers for all of your doctors
- List of all medical conditions you have (include any surgeries you have had)
- List of allergies for each household member
- List of medications taken by each household member

- Medical consent forms for each household member. These forms will allow someone to authorize medical treatment in an emergency situation when you're unable to give consent. Ask your physician or insurance company for information on how to obtain these forms.

Medicines and Supplies

- Antacid
- Antibiotic cream or ointment
- Antidiarrhea medication
- Antiseptic lotion or spray
- Calamine lotion (for rashes or itching)
- Disposable, instant-activating cold packs for icing injuries and burns
- Eyewash and eyepatch
- Flashlight
- Ipecac (to induce vomiting)
- Large gauze pads (to apply pressure to a large bleeding wound)
- Latex gloves
- Moistened sterile towelettes
- Needle

- Pain/fever medication, such as aspirin or acetaminophen
- Petroleum jelly or other lubricant
- Rubbing alcohol or hydrogen peroxide
- Safety pins
- Scissors
- Soap
- Square cloth of sufficient size to use as a sling
- Sterile adhesive bandages, gauze pads (four-by-four-inch or two-by-two-inch), adhesive tape
- Thermal blanket
- Thermometer
- Tongue depressors
- Tweezers

Anaphylaxis (Severe Allergic Reaction)

A<small>N</small> allergic reaction is a sensitivity to a specific substance, or *allergen.* You can come in contact with the allergen by touching, breathing, or swallowing it. The allergen can also be injected into your body. Common allergens include plants, foods, medications (especially penicillin), pollens, and venom from insect stings or bites.

Most allergic reactions are mild. But some people can have a severe reaction that can cause breathing problems and a dangerous drop in blood pressure *(anaphylactic shock).* Without medical intervention, this reaction can lead to death within 15 minutes.

What to Do

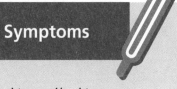

Symptoms

- Itching and/or hives
- Warm skin or flushed face
- Dizziness
- Swollen face or tongue
- Wheezing
- Nausea or vomiting
- Abdominal cramps
- Difficulty breathing
- Unconsciousness

1. **Call immediately for emergency medical assistance if the allergic reaction is severe or rapidly worsening or if the victim has a history of severe allergic reactions (check for a medical alert tag).**

2. If the person has emergency allergy medication nearby, such as an EpiPen®, help with the injection or inhalation of the medication.

3. Calm and reassure the person that help is on the way.

4. Do the ABCs of CPR (pp. 298-300). Check the person's airway, breathing, and circulation (pulse). If necessary, begin chest compression and rescue breathing.

5. Try to identify the allergen. If it is a bee sting, use a fingernail, a credit card, or other stiff material to scrape the stinger off the skin. Do not use tweezers, and don't squeeze the stinger; such actions will release more venom.

6. Help prevent **shock** (p. 317).

Bleeding

When to Seek Help

• If the bleeding doesn't stop after five minutes	▶ *Seek emergency care immediately.*
• If blood is spurting or gushing	▶ *Seek emergency care immediately.*

What to Do for Severe Bleeding

1. **Call 911 or go to an emergency room immediately.**

2. Do not move the person unless absolutely necessary if you suspect a head, neck, or back injury.

3. While waiting for help, apply firm, constant pressure to the wound with a clean cloth. If the cloth becomes soaked with blood, place a new one on top of it and continue pressing. Do not remove used dressings.

4. If a foreign object (such as glass) is in the wound, apply pressure alongside it, not on top of it. Do not remove the object.

5. Make the person as comfortable as possible. Elevate the part of the body that's bleeding so that it is higher than the heart, if possible. This will help reduce blood flow.

What to Do for Minor Bleeding from a Cut or Wound

1. Clean the wound with soap and water.

2. Blot the wound dry with sterile gauze or cloth.

3. Apply gentle pressure to stop bleeding.

4. Once bleeding has stopped, apply a bandage. For a puncture wound, apply an antiseptic solution to the wound and cover it with a sterile gauze pad. Avoid taping a puncture wound closed; sealing it increases the risk of infection.

5. Watch the wound for signs of infection—an increase in redness, swelling, pain, or discharge. If these signs appear, call your doctor.

ARE YOU DUE FOR ANOTHER TETANUS SHOT?

Tetanus is a painful and life-threatening illness that strikes the nervous system. It is contracted when bacteria invades an open wound, usually a deep puncture or cut.

Vaccines have made tetanus very rare in the United States. The illness strikes only about 40 to 60 people each year. Most of those cases involve people over the age of 50—people who either were never vaccinated against tetanus or have lost their immunity to it. Studies have shown that more than 70 percent of people aged 60 and older are no longer immune to the illness. You should have a tetanus booster every 10 years or as recommended by your physician. If you don't know when you last had a tetanus shot, ask your doctor.

Broken Bones

What to Do

1. **Call immediately for emergency medical assistance if the person shows symptoms of shock (p. 317) or if he or she is unconscious or cannot be moved.**

2. If you suspect an injury to the head, neck, back, hip, pelvis, or upper leg, do not move the person unless absolutely necessary.

3. Calm and reassure the person that help is on the way.

4. Do the ABCs of CPR (pp. 298-300). Check the person's airway, breathing, and circulation (pulse). If necessary, begin chest compression and rescue breathing.

5. Check for and treat any other serious injuries, such as **bleeding** (p. 304). Also, treat for **shock** (p. 317), if necessary.

6. Immobilize the injured bone or joint with a splint. Place soft material around the injury. Then attach a stiff object (such as a board, piece of cardboard, or rolled-up magazine or newspaper) to the injured limb. Fasten the splint with a rope, belt, or strips of cloth. Do not tie the splint in place directly over the break in the bone. Also, do not fasten too tightly. Never try to bend a displaced bone back in place or straighten an injured leg or hip that seems oddly positioned.

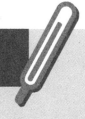

Symptoms

- Pain that worsens with movement
- Tenderness to the touch, or severe pain, especially in one spot
- Misshapen body part
- Swelling or bruising
- Discolored skin
- Numbness in arm or leg

Broken hip

- Pain in the hip, lower back, or groin area
- Pain in these areas that worsens with movement of the leg

Burns

When to Seek Help

- If the person is a child or elderly ▶ *Seek emergency care immediately.*

- If burn covers more than one body part ▶ *Seek emergency care immediately.*

- If burn is located on any sensitive area of the body, such as hands, face, or feet ▶ *Seek emergency care immediately.*

- If burn is third-degree (p. 308) ▶ *Seek emergency care immediately.*

- If burn is caused by chemicals or electricity ▶ *Seek emergency care immediately.*

- If burn involves inhalation ▶ *Seek emergency care immediately.*

Third-Degree Burns

Third-degree burns go through all the layers of the skin.

What to Do

1. **Seek emergency care as soon as possible.**

2. Do not remove any clothing near or at the site of the burn.

3. Do not apply cold water or medication to the burn.

4. If burns are on arms or legs, keep the limbs elevated above the level of the heart.

5. If person has burns on face, check frequently to make sure he or she is not having difficulty breathing.

Symptoms

Third-Degree Burns

- Skin looks whitish or charred

- Skin may break open, revealing underlying muscle or tendons

- Severe pain or, if nerves have been damaged, no pain except around edges of burn

Second-Degree Burns

Second-degree burns go through to the second layer of skin.

What to Do

1. Immerse the burned area of skin in cold water or place cold, wet cloths on it immediately.

2. Gently blot the area dry. Do not rub. Rubbing may break the blister, opening it to infection.

3. Cover the wound with a dry, sterile bandage.

4. If burn is located on an arm or leg, raise the limb as much as possible; this will help reduce swelling.

5. Call your doctor as soon as possible.

Symptoms

Second-Degree Burns

- Blisters

- Rough, red skin

- Swelling

First-Degree Burns

First-degree burns affect only the outer layer of skin, but they can be very painful.

What to Do

1. Immediately immerse the burned area of skin in cold water.

2. Run cool water over the burn, or place cold, wet cloths on it, for about 10 minutes or until the pain decreases.

3. Cover the burn with a sterile bandage or clean cloth.

4. Take aspirin or acetaminophen to relieve any pain or swelling.

5. If the burn fails to heal over the next few days, call your doctor.

Chemical Burns

What to Do

1. **Seek emergency care as soon as possible.**

2. Move the person away from the chemical.

3. Brush off any dry chemicals. (Be sure to protect your hands with gloves or clothing.)

4. Remove clothing on or near the burn area. Never pull clothing over the head with a chemical burn. You may need to cut the clothing.

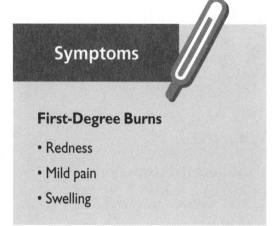

Symptoms

First-Degree Burns

• Redness

• Mild pain

• Swelling

Symptoms

Chemical Burns

• Burn marks or blisters

• Headache or stomach pain

• Breathing problems

• Seizures or dizziness

• Loss of consciousness

5. Wash the area thoroughly with running water for at least 20 minutes.

6. If the burn is in the eye, wash from the inside corner to the outside of the open eye.

7. Cover the burn with a clean, dry cloth.

Choking

What to Do

If the person is conscious:

1. Ask, "Are you choking?" If the person can speak, cough, or breathe, do not interfere. **WARNING: Never slap a person on the back if he or she is coughing effectively.** The slap may cause the person to inhale the object, which may result in complete blockage of the windpipe.

2. **If the person cannot speak, cough, or breathe, or is making a high-pitched wheezing sound, call 911 immediately.** Then give abdominal thrusts (the Heimlich maneuver—see opposite).

3. Continue giving abdominal thrusts until the object is dislodged or emergency care arrives.

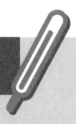

Symptoms

- High-pitched wheezing
- Universal distress sign—grabbing at the throat
- Inability to speak, cough forcefully, or breathe
- Bluish face
- Loss of consciousness

CAUTION

Anyone who has been rescued from a choking episode should see a doctor. The abdominal thrusts needed to dislodge the object may have damaged the chest or abdomen. Also, the trapped object may have damaged the throat.

The Heimlich Maneuver

1. Stand behind the person and place your arms around his or her waist.

2. With one hand, make a fist and place it, thumb side first, against the person's stomach slightly above the navel.

3. Grasp your fist with your other hand and press into the person's stomach with a quick upward thrust.

4. Repeat up to six times to clear the airway.

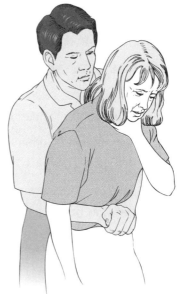

If You Are Choking and Alone

1. Give yourself abdominal thrusts. Make a fist and place it against your stomach, slightly above the navel. Use your other hand to thrust your fist up and into your abdomen.

2. You can also use the back of a chair or a railing. Lean forward and press your abdomen against it.

continued on next page

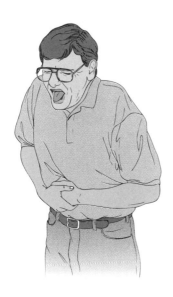

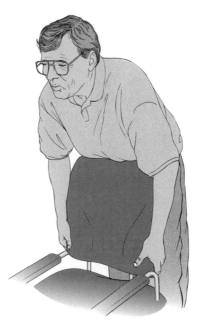

If the person becomes unconscious:

1. Lay the person on his or her back.

2. Open the person's mouth.

3. Using your finger, sweep deep inside the person's mouth to remove any blockage.*
   Be careful not to push any object deeper into the throat.

4. Tilt the person's head back and lift his or her chin. Put your ear to the person's
   mouth to listen for breathing.

5. If the person is not breathing, begin rescue breaths. Pinch the person's nose and
   give two slow breaths into his or her mouth. If the chest does not move, tilt the
   head back further and repeat the breaths.

6. If chest still does not rise, give up to five abdominal thrusts. To do this, straddle
   your legs across the person's thighs. Place the heel of one hand over the person's
   stomach area. Cover it with your other hand. Keep both arms straight and press
   into the stomach with a quick inward and upward thrust.

7. Repeat steps 4 through 6 until successful.

8. After the obstruction is removed, begin the ABCs of CPR, if necessary (pp. 298-300).

*NOTE: The American Heart Association (AHA) is in the process of revising this step
in their CPR procedure. For more information, contact the AHA (p. 345).

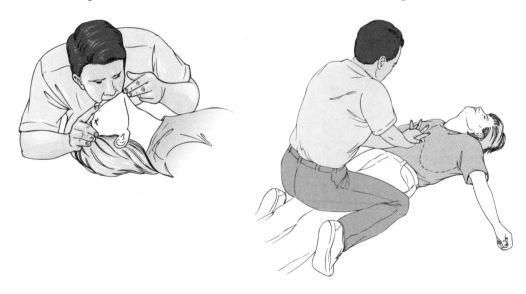

Heatstroke and Heat Exhaustion

HEATSTROKE and heat exhaustion can strike people of all ages but are most common in older people. People with preexisting medical conditions, such as **diabetes** or blood vessel disease, are also more susceptible to heat illnesses. That's because many illnesses—and the medications used to treat them—can interfere with how the body dissipates heat.

Learn the symptoms of heat exhaustion. Take immediate action if you or anyone you know has these symptoms. Heat exhaustion can quickly lead to heatstroke, a life-threatening condition that requires emergency intervention.

Symptoms

Heatstroke

- Hot, dry, flushed skin
- No sweating
- Rapid heartbeat
- Nausea or vomiting
- High body temperature
- Confusion
- Loss of consciousness
- Extreme weakness
- Seizures

Heat Exhaustion

- Painful muscle cramps
- Cool, moist, pale skin
- Weakness
- Headache
- Fast, shallow breathing
- Heavy sweating
- Intense thirst

What to Do

Heatstroke

1. **If you suspect the person has heatstroke, call for emergency medical help immediately.**

2. While waiting for help to arrive, follow the steps for heat exhaustion below.

Heat Exhaustion

1. Have the person lie down in a cool place, with his or her legs elevated.

2. Cool the person rapidly. Loosen tight clothing. Place cool, wet cloths on the person's face and body, or wrap the person in wet sheets. Also, fan the person with an electric fan, a hair dryer set on cool, or your hand.

3. If the person is fully awake, give him or her a cool drink.

4. Call for emergency medical help if the person's condition does not improve.

Hypothermia and Frostbite

As we age, we lose some of our body's subcutaneous fat, our natural insulation that protects us against cold. We are also more likely to have illnesses or take medications that impede the body's ability to regulate its temperature. These are major reasons we tend to complain of feeling cold when we are older—and why we are at greater risk of developing hypothermia and frostbite.

Hypothermia occurs when body temperature drops below normal and the body begins to lose heat faster than it can produce it. If untreated, this condition can develop into a serious, even life-threatening, health problem quite quickly. In severe cases, hypothermia can cause the heart to beat irregularly, which may lead to heart failure and death.

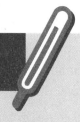

Symptoms

Hypothermia

- Constant shivering
- Urge to urinate
- Muscle stiffness
- Weak pulse
- Confusion or sleepiness
- Slowed, slurred speech

Frostbite

- White or yellowish skin
- Skin that itches or burns
- Numb, reddened, or swollen skin
- Skin that feels unusually firm or waxy

Frostbite is the freezing of body tissue, usually skin. About 90 percent of cases involve the feet and hands. Older people, especially those with circulatory problems, are at increased risk of developing this problem.

You do not need below-freezing temperatures to experience either hypothermia or frostbite. Both can occur in mildly cool temperatures as well, particularly when it is windy or wet.

What to Do

Hypothermia

1. **Call for emergency medical care immediately.**

2. Do the ABCs of CPR (pp. 298-300). Check the person's airway, breathing, and circulation (pulse). If necessary, begin chest compression and rescue breathing.

3. If medical help is unavailable, begin warming the person. If possible, get the victim into a warm room or shelter. If the person has on any wet clothing, remove it.

4. Warm the center of the body first—chest, neck, head, and groin—using warm compresses or an electric blanket, if available. Or use skin-to-skin contact under loose, dry layers of blankets, clothing, towels, or sheets.

5. If the person is awake and can swallow, give him or her warm beverages. Do not give alcoholic beverages.

6. After body temperature has increased, keep the person dry and wrapped in a warm blanket, including the head and neck.

7. Get medical attention as soon as possible.

Frostbite

1. **Call for emergency medical care.**

2. Get the person into a warm room. Remove tight clothing and jewelry.

3. Unless absolutely necessary, do not let the person walk on frostbitten feet or toes. This increases the damage.

4. If help will not arrive soon, slowly thaw the frostbitten skin. Apply warm moist compresses or submerge the affected area in warm—not hot—water. (The temperature should be comfortable to the touch.)

5. Do not rub frostbitten areas or apply direct heat. Frostbitten skin must be warmed slowly to prevent permanent damage.

Shock

SHOCK happens when there is a sudden, severe loss of blood or other body fluids. It can be caused by a wound or by an illness. Shock requires medical treatment to be reversed. All you can do is help prevent it from getting worse.

What to Do

1. **Call for emergency medical help immediately.**

2. Do not move the person unless absolutely necessary if you suspect a head, neck, or back injury.

3. Do the ABCs of CPR (pp. 298-300). Check the person's airway, breathing, and circulation (pulse). If necessary, begin chest compression and rescue breathing.

4. Make the person comfortable. Lay the person on his or her back, unless you suspect a head, neck, or back injury. Keep the person's feet elevated about 12 inches above the heart if possible. Do not elevate the person's head.

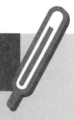

Symptoms

- Bluish skin, lips, or fingernails
- Cool, clammy skin
- Dull and sunken eyes
- Chills and shakiness
- Weak, rapid pulse
- Rapid, shallow breathing
- Nausea or vomiting
- Unusual thirst
- Unconsciousness

5. Keep the person warm, unless the cause of the shock is heatstroke (p. 313).

6. Do not give the person anything to eat or drink.

7. Try to determine the cause of shock. Check for a medical alert tag. Ask the person or bystanders what happened.

8. Monitor the person. If the person begins to vomit, turn his or her head to one side to allow fluid to drain out.

Staying Safe

As we age, we become more prone to accidental injuries, especially from falls, fires, and automobile accidents. Thousands of older people die from such injuries each year. Many more thousands become permanently disabled, their lives forever altered. They suddenly find themselves with decreased mobility, a more restricted lifestyle, and increased dependence on others for their day-to-day needs.

With age, we also become more vulnerable to crime, whether at the hands of strangers or of people we know. When we become the victims of crime, we can suffer both psychological as well as physical injuries. Such injuries can have a major impact on our health and our lifestyle. Some types of crime also can deal a devastating financial blow from which we may find it difficult to recover.

You can do many things to protect your safety and lower your risk of becoming a victim of an accident or a crime. Prevention is the key to staying safe, as you'll discover as you read the following pages.

Preventing Falls

As you age, your risk of falling increases. About 30 percent of people over age 65 fall each year. The risk of a hip fracture—one of the most disabling fall-related injuries—doubles every five to six years after age 50.

Most falls do not result in broken bones or other serious injury. But, unfortunately, many do. Such injuries can lead to permanent disabilities and a decline in health. They can also greatly limit your movement—and your daily activities.

Older people are more prone to falling for a number of reasons. As we age, our reaction times slow and our sense of balance declines. Age-related **vision problems**, such as cataracts and glaucoma, also can affect our perception and coordination. So can other conditions and illnesses that often strike older people, such as **stroke**, **Parkinson's disease**, and **arthritis**. In addition, older people tend to take more medications. Many drugs, including diuretics, sedatives, and those for **high blood pressure**, can lead to balance problems.

Inactivity is another important factor in why so many older people fall. If you don't stay physically active, you lose some of your muscle conditioning and balance. This increases your risk of falling.

Tips for Staying on Your Feet

- Exercise. It can build muscle tone, strengthen bones, and improve your balance.

- Have your vision and hearing checked regularly.

- Talk to your doctor or pharmacist about side effects of drugs that could affect your coordination and balance.

- Make your home safer. (See suggestions, opposite.)

- Limit the amount of alcohol you drink. It affects balance and slows reaction time.

- Walk cautiously. You can test surfaces by moving your foot back and forth on them.

- Be especially careful when walking outdoors on wet or icy sidewalks.

- During winter, use salt and sand liberally on sidewalks, steps, and driveways. And remember: Melted snow can refreeze overnight into ice.

- If you are concerned about falling, ask someone to assist you.

Make Your Home Safer

About half of all falls happen at home. To make your home safer:

- Remove things you can trip over (such as papers, books, clothes, and shoes) from stairs and places where you walk.

- Remove small throw rugs or use double-sided tape to keep the rugs from slipping.

- Keep items you use often in cabinets you can reach easily without using a step stool.

- Have grab bars put in next to your toilet and in the tub or shower.

- Use nonslip mats in the bathtub and on shower floors.

- Improve the lighting in your home. As you get older, you need brighter lights to see well. Lamp shades or frosted bulbs can reduce glare.

- Have handrails and lights put in on all staircases.

- Wear shoes that give good support and have thin, nonslip soles. Avoid wearing slippers and athletic shoes with deep treads.

Source: National Center for Injury Prevention and Control

IF YOU FALL

- Stay calm. Determine whether you are hurt.

- If you can, crawl along the floor to the nearest sturdy chair and try to get up.

- If you can't pull yourself up, shout for help.

- If you are alone, crawl slowly to the telephone. Call 911 or someone (perhaps a relative or a friend) who can come and help you.

Preventing Fires and Burns

OLDER people are one of the groups at greatest risk of dying in a fire. Each year, fires claim the lives of about 1,200 Americans over the age of 65. The older we get, the greater the risk. Once we pass the age of 80, we are three times more likely than the rest of the population to die as the result of fire-related injuries.

Why the increased risk? As we age, we become less able to move and act quickly when a fire breaks out—a slowness that may be enhanced by illness or medications. In addition, many older people live alone, with no one to help out in an emergency.

The leading causes of fire-related injuries and deaths among older people are smoking and cooking accidents, heating equipment, and faulty wiring. Fortunately, you can take a number of preventive steps to dramatically reduce your chances of becoming the victim of a fire.

Fire Prevention Tips

- Install at least one smoke detector outside every bedroom (or inside, if you sleep with your bedroom door closed) and on every level of your house. Check the batteries in the detectors monthly. Replace them at least once a year. Many people replace them twice a year on the same day they set their clocks backward or forward.

- Have a sound fire escape plan. Plan and practice the route. Make sure everyone in your family knows two ways out of every room.

- Never leave smoking materials or candles unattended. Empty all ashtrays into the toilet or a metal container every night before going to bed. Never smoke in bed. Better yet, quit smoking altogether.

- Never leave food unattended on the stove or in the oven. If you must leave the kitchen briefly, take a spoon or a potholder with you to remind you to return.

- Keep items away from the stove that could catch fire, such as towels, curtains, and plastic. Also, never cook wearing clothes with loose, dangling sleeves.

WHAT TO DO WHEN A FIRE BREAKS OUT

Every member of your family should know the following steps to take in case of fire:

- Get out of the house as quickly as possible. Don't stop to try to save valuables.

- If you can safely do so, close the door of the room where the fire has started and close all other doors behind you. This will help delay the spread of smoke.

- Crawl low, under the smoke. Cover your mouth and nose with a piece of cloth. Most fire victims die from smoke inhalation and lack of oxygen.

- Touch closed doors with the back of your hand before opening them. Never open a door that feels warm.

- Never return to a burning house.

- Call 911 after you've left a burning building. Do not call from inside.

- If clothes catch on fire, "stop, drop, and roll" to extinguish the flames.

- Keep a fire extinguisher in the kitchen. Make sure you know how to use it.

- If you have a portable heater, keep it away from blankets, clothing, curtains, furniture, or anything else that could get hot and catch fire.

- Plug portable heaters directly into a wall socket. Unplug them when they are not in use.

- Make sure the electrical wiring in your home is up to code.

- Avoid overloading electrical outlets. Don't run cords under carpets or furniture.

Preventing Auto Accidents

Y OU can be a poor or great driver at any age. Generally speaking, however, driving skills begin to decline at about age 55, with the drop being especially dramatic after age 75. In fact, people aged 85 and older have a crash rate higher than teenagers. They are also nine times more likely to die in an automobile crash than someone aged 25 to 69.

Why do our driving skills decline as we get older? Reduced vision, particularly at night, is a major factor. Age also affects our depth perception and our peripheral vision, making left-hand turns and lane changes more difficult to maneuver. In addition, certain conditions associated with aging, such as **arthritis** and **Parkinson's disease**, can impede our ability to control a car. And, finally, older people tend to take more medications. Many of these drugs have side effects—blurred vision, increased drowsiness, reduced concentration—that can affect driving.

Fortunately, there are many things you can do to help compensate for the effects of aging and improve your driving safety.

Safe Driving Tips

- Have regular vision and hearing tests.
- Avoid driving during heavy traffic and bad weather.
- If night vision is a problem, limit your driving to daytime hours.
- Avoid driving for long periods of time. Stop and stretch often.
- Be especially careful when pulling out into traffic. Because peripheral vision decreases with age, you'll need to turn your head farther to see what's around your car.
- Have a wide rearview mirror installed in your car. Check all your mirrors frequently.
- Avoid driving in cars with heavily tinted windshields and windows. Also, don't wear tinted glasses or sunglasses when driving in low light.
- Keep your windshield clean, inside as well as outside.

- Leave a three-second safety cushion between you and the car in front of you. Remember: Your reaction time is probably slower than when you were younger.

- Plan your route ahead of time. You can then concentrate on driving rather than on navigating.

- Ask passengers to help you navigate.

- Check with your doctor about the side effects of any medications you are taking.

- Take a driver refresher course. Such courses are offered by AARP, the Automobile Association of America (AAA), the National Safety Council, and others. Some insurance companies offer discounts to older drivers who complete a refresher course.

- Listen to your family and friends if they have any concerns about your driving. To reassure them (and yourself), have your driving skills evaluated at a local rehabilitation center or state licensing agency.

Self-Test

Should You Still Be Driving?

Do you have difficulty seeing pedestrians, objects, and other vehicles?
❑ Yes   ❑ No

Do you find it difficult to coordinate hand and foot movements?
❑ Yes   ❑ No

Do you sense that the traffic is moving too quickly around you?
❑ Yes   ❑ No

Are other drivers always honking their horns at you?
❑ Yes   ❑ No

Do cars seem to appear from nowhere when you're driving?
❑ Yes   ❑ No

Have you unintentionally run stop signs or red lights?
❑ Yes   ❑ No

Have you found yourself getting lost while driving in familiar areas?
❑ Yes   ❑ No

Are your family members or friends expressing real concern about your driving?
❑ Yes   ❑ No

If you answered "yes" to any of these questions, it may be time for you to stop driving.

A Difficult Decision

Being able to drive means so much more than simply being able to get from point A to point B. Driving provides us with easy access to friends, family, employment, shopping, educational and cultural experiences, and so much more. It also enables us to be self-sufficient and independent.

No wonder so many of us resist the idea of hanging up our car keys for good. We know the effect it will have on our daily lives.

But continuing to drive when it's no longer safe for you to do so can also have a serious impact on your life. Chances are you will eventually have an accident that will injure either you or someone else. The repercussions of such an accident can be devastating, both physically and emotionally.

You can take several steps to make the transition to not driving easier. First, talk with your family and friends. They may be quite ready to help you get to many of the places you need to go, such as the grocery store or the doctor's office. You can also use taxis, buses, and other forms of public transportation. Many communities offer low-fee door-to-door van service for older people. Your local senior citizen center should be able to help you connect with these services.

Finally, some older people opt to keep their automobiles after they stop driving. When they need to get someplace, they simply hand the keys to someone else.

Preventing Crime

HERE'S the good news: As we get older, it becomes statistically less likely that we will become the victim of a crime.

Now the bad news: Even so, about two million older people become crime victims each year.

People over the age of 50 are particularly vulnerable to crimes such as burglary, robbery, and fraud—often with devastating effects. Older people are more likely than younger people to suffer serious physical harm during a crime. And because older people are more susceptible to financial fraud, they are more likely to lose a significant amount of money—and suffer a drop in their standard of living—as a result of a crime.

Attacks by strangers are more common among older people than among younger people. But it isn't only strangers who commit crimes against older people. Sometimes family members, friends, or caretakers abuse older people, either through neglect, through violence, or by stealing money or property. In addition to learning how to protect yourself against stranger crime, be sure you also take steps to protect yourself against criminal acts from people you know. (See "Preventing Abuse and Neglect," pp. 330-331.)

Crime Prevention Tips

Don't let fear of crime stop you from enjoying life. You can do many things to protect yourself without curtailing your daily activities.

At Home

- Never open your door before knowing who's there. Look through a peephole or a safe window.

- Lock your doors and windows. Also, lock your garage.

- Vary your daily routine.

- Keep an inventory of all expensive items in your home, such as jewelry, silver, and antiques. Also, take pictures of these items. Store the inventory and pictures in a safe place, like a bank safety deposit box.

- When you are away from your home, make it look as if it is still occupied. Leave the radio or TV on. Use an automatic timer to turn lights on at night. Making an empty house look occupied is especially important if you will be gone for more than a day.

- Keep your home well lit at night, inside and out; keep curtains closed.

- Never let a stranger into your house. Ask for proper identification from delivery or repair people. If you feel worried, call the company to verify. If a stranger comes to your door and asks to use your phone, offer to place the call yourself.

- Form a "neighborhood watch" with your neighbors. A concerned neighbor who will report suspicious persons and activities promptly to the police is often the best protection against crime.

Away from Home

- Stay alert at all times. Pay attention when walking or driving; notice who's around you.

- Whether walking or driving, plan your route ahead of time.

- Carry a cell phone; keep it regularly charged.

- Try to stay away from places where crimes happen, such as dark parking lots or alleys.

- Have a friend accompany you whenever possible.

- Carry your purse close to your body. Put a wallet in an inside coat or front pants pocket.

- Avoid carrying credit cards you don't need or large amounts of cash.

- Have your monthly pension or Social Security checks sent direct-deposit, right to your bank. If you visit the bank often, vary the time of day you go.

- Havc your keys ready when approaching your car or front door.

- When in a car, keep your door locked.

- Sit close to the driver or near the exit while riding in a bus, train, or subway.

- If someone is making you feel uneasy, trust your instincts and leave.

- Carry a whistle or other alarm device and keep it accessible.

WATCH OUT FOR CON ARTISTS

Older people are favorite targets of fraudulent telemarketers and other con artists. Protect yourself by following these tips from the FBI:

- Be skeptical of offers that sound "too good to be true." They usually are.

- Resist high-pressure sales tactics. Don't allow yourself to be hurried into a decision.

- Never give your credit card number or checking account information to anyone over the telephone unless you know whom you are dealing with.

- Don't spend or invest more than you can afford to lose.

- Companies should be willing to provide their name, address, phone number, and references. If they're not, be skeptical. Verify this information before making a purchase.

- If you are skeptical about a company, check with the Better Business Bureau before you make a purchase.

- Report incidents of telemarketing fraud to your local Better Business Bureau or your local law enforcement authority.

- Never let anyone else use your bank card. Never give anyone your personal identification number (PIN).

Preventing Abuse and Neglect

THE abuse and neglect of older people—sometimes referred to as "elder abuse"—is a significant problem. Experts estimate that up to two million Americans are victims of elder abuse every year.

Most cases are never reported, however. Older people who are being abused often fear going to authorities; they worry that the abuser will retaliate or that they themselves will be taken out of their home and institutionalized. Some feel too ashamed to report the abuse, particularly if the abuser is a family member. Many older people simply do not know where to seek help; they may live alone or with their abuser and have little or no contact with others in their communities. Or they may have mental or physical disabilities, caused by such illnesses as **Alzheimer's disease** or **stroke**, that make it impossible for them to communicate effectively or leave home to get help.

Abuse can happen to anyone. But it doesn't need to keep happening. In recent years elder abuse has become recognized as a serious problem. There are now many places to go for help. If you think you are being abused in any way, or if you think someone you know is being abused, get help now.

Common Types of Elder Abuse

- Physical abuse. This type of abuse occurs when someone hits or slaps you, sexually assaults you, deprives you of food or water, or inflicts some other form of physical pain or injury.

- Emotional abuse. This type of abuse occurs when someone calls you names, harasses you, or humiliates, intimidates, or threatens you.

- Financial abuse. This type of abuse occurs when someone steals or misuses your belongings or your money.

Prevention

- Stay connected with people. The wider your network of friends, the less likely it is that someone will take advantage of you. When you move, keep in contact with old friends and neighbors. Talk regularly with them. Invite them to visit you. Be sure to make new friends as well.

- Remain active. Join a group or organization. Sign up for a class. Volunteer. Also, set up and keep regular medical, dental, or beauty appointments.

- Keep organized. Know where you keep everything, especially your valuables and financial papers. Open and post your own mail.

- Purchase an answering machine and use it to screen calls. An answering machine can help you avoid unscrupulous telemarketers.

- Always get legal advice before agreeing to new financial arrangements, such as powers of attorney for health and finances. Never sign a document unless your lawyer or someone you trust has reviewed it. Review your will periodically.

- Know where you can go for help should you become the victim of elder abuse.

Where to Go for Help

- **If you are in immediate fear of your physical safety, call 911.**

- The National Center on Elder Abuse (NCEA) can help put you in contact with adult protective service agencies in your area. Call the NCEA Eldercare Locator: 1-800-677-1116.

- You can also tell your doctor, who will assist you in getting help.

- At the very least, talk to a trusted friend or relative. Ask that person to get help for you.

Looking Ahead

Chances are, you'll stay independent most of your life. But late in life—when you reach your 80s or 90s—you may begin to need help with everyday tasks, such as shopping, cooking, taking medication, walking, or bathing. Even at an earlier age, an illness or accident may make it necessary for you to have help. That help may come from family or friends. Or it may come from professionals, either in your home or in a nursing home or other long-term care facility.

It's important that you plan for those years now. Planning can help you stay independent longer. It also can help you and your family make wiser decisions—*before* a crisis strikes.

Are You Financially Fit?

Experts estimate that you'll need at least 70 percent of your preretirement income to maintain your standard of living when you retire. Social Security pays the average retiree about 40 percent of preretirement earnings. You'll need to make up the 30 percent difference from your pension and savings. You may even need to continue earning income from part-time employment.

Unfortunately, less than half of Americans have put aside money specifically for retirement. That means they may not be able to afford the lifestyle they had hoped for in their later years. But whether your retirement is months or years away, it is never too late to start planning for it. And even if you are already retired, you may be able to take some steps to improve your financial situation.

Here are tips for retirement planning:

- Know your retirement needs. Calculate how much money you'll need to maintain a reasonable standard of living in retirement. Remember, the experts say it will be at least 70 percent of your preretirement income.

- Find out about your Social Security benefits. The Social Security Administration can give you an estimate of how much your benefits will be when you retire. Call them at 1-800-772-1213 and ask for a Personal Earnings and Benefit Estimate Statement. It's free.

- Find out what your pension or profit-sharing plan through your employer is worth. Most employers will give you an individual benefit statement if you ask for one. Also, learn what benefits you may have from previous jobs. And find out if you will be entitled to benefits from your spouse's plan.

- Start saving now to fill the gap between what Social Security, your pension, and existing savings will earn you in retirement and what you will need to maintain a reasonable standard of living. Make saving for retirement a high priority. Set goals and stick to them.

Tips for Getting Your Financial Papers in Order

It's important to get your financial papers in order in case you become ill or disabled. Here are some suggestions:

- Make a list of all your important financial and legal documents. Note where they are kept or stored. Include information on bank and brokerage statements, credit cards, income tax records, insurance policies, property tax receipts, pension records, and your will.

- Make a list of the names, phone numbers, and addresses of all the professional people who are involved in your affairs. Include your physicians, dentist, clergy, attorney, accountant, insurance agent, banker, and financial adviser.

- Make a list of the names, phone numbers, and addresses of all people who should be notified if you become incapacitated or die. Include your children, parents, closest relatives or friends, and the people named in your will.

- Make sure the person you have designated to take care of your financial affairs if you become incapacitated or die has easy access to all of the above documents.

- Arrange automatic payment of as many of your recurring bills as possible (such as your water, electric and other utilities, health insurance, and mortgage bills). This will make it easier for the person who will be managing your financial affairs should you become ill or disabled. It also will help ensure that you won't experience any interruptions in service while you are in a hospital.

- Have any income you receive—such as Social Security checks, pension checks, and stock dividends—automatically deposited into your bank account.

Consider Setting Up a "Durable Power of Attorney"

A durable power of attorney is a legal document in which you give one or more people the authority to handle your finances, property, or other personal matters if you should become incapacitated. It is a simple and inexpensive way to make sure that your financial affairs are handled according to your wishes.

If you do not set up a durable power of attorney, you will have to hope that a relative or friend will step forward and volunteer to manage your financial affairs. This person will have to go before a judge to be appointed conservator, or guardian of your estate. This can be a time-consuming and costly proceeding.

Even if you are married or have put most of your property into a living trust, setting up a durable power of attorney is often a wise idea. It's a simple process. All you need to do is sign a single legal document that names the person you wish to be your agent. No court hearing is required. The document must be signed in front of a notary public, however, and in some states witnesses also must be present when you sign it. Although not required, it is best to consult an attorney before signing a durable power of attorney.

A durable power of attorney can be drafted so that it goes into effect as soon as you sign it. But you can also specify that it go into effect only after a doctor certifies that you have become incapacitated. In addition, you can have the document drafted to give your agent as much or as little power over your financial affairs as you like. And you can revoke the document at any time as long as you are mentally competent.

Advance Directives

Once you become seriously ill or injured, you may become so incapacitated that decisions about your health care may be out of your control. With an advance directive, however, you can make sure your preferences for medical treatment are carried out, even if you are unable to speak for yourself.

There are two basic types of advance directives: a living will and a health care power of attorney. Both are legal documents. In a living will, you put in writing what you do—and don't—want done for you medically in the event that you become terminally ill or near death and cannot speak for yourself. Each state has different laws governing living wills. Some, for example, limit the treatments to which the living will applies.

A health care power of attorney is a legal document in which you identify someone to make decisions about your medical treatment when you are no longer able to make those decisions yourself. It is *not* the same as a durable power of attorney, a document in which you designate someone to take care of your financial affairs (see p. 335).

In some states, doctors are allowed to choose a "proxy decision maker" for you if you don't have an advance directive. Usually, these laws instruct the doctors to turn first to a spouse for guidance, then to an adult child, and then to a parent or an adult brother or sister. If you do not want these people, in this order, making health care decisions for you, then it's crucial that you fill out a health care power of attorney.

For more information about advance directives, talk to your physician or your attorney. You can also call the aging or health services departments in your state.

Housing Options

Most of us, when asked, say we want to stay in our own home for as long as possible. Our homes evoke warm memories. They also represent security and independence.

Yet as we grow older, caring for a home can become difficult. Tasks we once performed quite easily—cooking, tending the garden, doing the laundry—may now exhaust us. Even tending to personal needs, such as bathing, may become problematic, if not impossible, as the result of an age-related illness or disability. Many people, of course, do find it possible to stay in their homes. They hire in-home services and caregivers to help them cope. For a fee, people will come to your home to cut your grass, do your shopping, cook your meals, and even take care of your personal care needs. This option can be expensive, however. It also requires considerable management, either by you or by a relative or friend.

At some point, you may need to relocate. Fortunately, many more housing options are available to older people today than in previous generations. These options can help you retain much of your independence for as long as possible.

Independent Living Retirement Communities

These communities are for older people who are able to live on their own but who want the convenience of certain basic services, such as meals, housekeeping, recreational activities, transportation, and security.

Assisted Living Facilities

These facilities bridge the gap between living independently and living in a nursing home. They offer an intermediate level of long-term care. In addition to the basic services of independent living retirement communities (opposite), assisted living facilities offer help with personal care. Residents can receive assistance in managing their medications, for example. They can also receive help with bathing, grooming, and dressing.

Assisted living facilities can be in a high-rise building or in a renovated Victorian house. They may house only a handful of residents or more than a hundred. Each resident devises an individual care plan when moving into the facility. The plan is then updated regularly.

Nursing Homes

These facilities are for people who require daily nursing care in addition to basic services. A skilled nursing facility is a nursing home that provides continuous (24-hour) nursing supervision by registered or licensed vocational nurses. An intermediate care facility (ICF) is required to provide only eight hours of nursing supervision each day. ICFs are for people who can move around on their own and who need limited nursing care.

Continuing Care Retirement Communities

These facilities offer different levels of care—independent, assisted living, and nursing home—at one site. Residents can then move from one type of care to another when necessary. This living arrangement can be especially helpful for couples when one of the spouses is disabled.

Group Homes

This type of living arrangement is sometimes called "sheltered" or "enriched" housing." It provides independent, private living in a house shared by several other older people. The costs of rent, housekeeping services, utilities, and meals are split among the residents. Group homes usually have a professional staff who help arrange services and social activities.

Finding the Right Place for You

Moving from a home into a new kind of living arrangement is a big change. You will have to adjust to a new setting, new friends—a new kind of lifestyle. Some facilities have social workers who can help you prepare for the change. You may also be able to get assistance from your local aging agency.

Here are some tips from the National Institute on Aging to help you find the residential program that's best for you. Start looking into these facilities long before you actually plan to make a move. That way, if you or your family needs to make a decision in a hurry—after a **stroke** or a hip fracture, for example—you will know what's available and affordable.

- Ask questions. Find out about specific facilities in your area. Doctors, friends and relatives, local hospital discharge planners and social workers, and religious organizations can help. Your state's office of the long-term care ombudsman has information about specific nursing homes and can let you know whether there have been problems at a particular home. Other types of residential arrangements don't follow the same federal, state, or local licensing requirements or regulations as nursing homes. Talk to people in your community or local social service agencies to find out which facilities seem to be well run.

- Call. Contact the places that interest you. Ask basic questions about vacancies, number of residents, costs and method of payment, and participation in Medicare and Medicaid. Also, think about what's important to you, such as transportation, meals, recreational activities, or medication policies.

- Visit. When you find a place that seems right, go talk to the staff, residents, and, if possible, family members of residents. Set up an appointment, but also go unannounced and at different times of the day. See if the staff treats residents with respect and tries to meet the needs of each person. Check whether the building is clean and safe. Are residents restrained in any way? Are social activities and exercise programs offered—and enjoyed? Do residents have personal privacy? Is the facility secure for people and their belongings? Eat a meal there to see if you like the food.

- Understand. Once you have made a choice, be sure you understand the facility's contract and financial agreement. It's a good idea to have a lawyer look them over before you sign.

Long-Term Care Insurance

You may never need the around-the-clock care of a nursing home. But the longer you live, the greater the chance that you will need some kind of long-term care. Such care can be very costly. Right now, a year in a nursing home is estimated to cost anywhere from $40,000 to $80,000. Having a nurse or home care aide come into your home is less expensive, but the cost can still run several thousand dollars a month.

Medicare covers very little of long-term care expenses. It is designed as an acute care program and therefore covers only hospital and physician expenses. Medicare does pay for some nursing home costs, but only on a limited basis—and usually following a hospital stay.

Medicaid will pay for long-term care services, but only after you have exhausted all your personal financial resources.

Medicare supplement insurance (often called Medigap or MedSupp) can fill in some of the gaps in Medicare coverage, such as hospital deductibles, doctors' deductibles, and coinsurance payments. But Medicare supplement insurance does not cover long-term care.

So how can you protect yourself and your family from the high costs of long-term medical care? For many people, private long-term care insurance is the answer. And unlike Medicaid, which focuses almost exclusively on institutional care, private long-term care insurance covers a wide range of services that can help people with illnesses or disabilities stay in their homes.

Buying a long-term medical care insurance policy is a complicated matter. Shop around. Contact several companies (and insurance agents) before you buy. Be sure you understand the policy completely before agreeing to it. And never let yourself be pressured or scared into making a quick decision.

The National Association of Insurance Commissioners has developed standards that protect consumers. They recommend that you look for a policy that includes the following:

- At least one year of nursing home or home health care coverage, including intermediate and custodial care. Nursing home or home health care benefits should not be limited primarily to skilled care.

- Coverage for **Alzheimer's disease**, should the policyholder develop it after purchasing the policy.

- An inflation protection option. The policy should offer a choice among 1) automatically increasing the initial benefit level on an annual basis, 2) a guaranteed right to increase benefit levels periodically without providing evidence of insurability, and 3) covering a specific percentage of actual or reasonable charges.

- An "outline of coverage" that systematically describes the policy's benefits, limitations, and exclusions and also allows you to compare it with others.

- A long-term care insurance shopper's guide that helps you decide whether long-term care insurance is appropriate for you.

- A guarantee that the policy cannot be canceled, made nonrenewable, or otherwise terminated because you get older or suffer deterioration in physical or mental health.

- The right to return the policy within 30 days after you have purchased it (if for any reason you do not want it) and to receive a premium refund.

- No requirement that policyholders first be hospitalized in order to receive nursing home benefits or home health care benefits, first receive skilled nursing home care before receiving intermediate or custodial nursing home care, or first receive nursing home care before receiving benefits for home health care.

Resources

AGING

Access America
Web site: www.seniors.gov
This comprehensive Web site is a joint effort by more than 16 federal agencies. Its purpose is to keep older people informed of services available on the Web.

AARP
601 E St. NW
Washington, DC 20049
1-800-424-3410
E-mail: member@aarp.org
Web site: www.AARP.org

American Geriatrics Society
The Empire State Building
350 Fifth Ave., Suite 801
New York, NY 10118
1-212-308-1414
E-mail: info@americangeriatrics.org
Web site: www.americangeriatrics.org

Leadership Council of Aging Organizations
Web site: www.lcao.org
A coalition of national nonprofit organizations concerned with the well-being of America's older population and committed to representing their interests in the policy-making arena.

National Association of State Units on Aging
1225 I St. NW, Suite 725
Washington, DC 20005
1-800-677-1116 (Eldercare Locator)
Web site:
www.aoa.dhhs.gov/aoa/dir/137.html

National Center on Elder Abuse
1225 I St. NW, Suite 725
Washington, DC 20005
1-202-898-2586
E-mail: NCEA@nasua.org
Web site: www.gwjapan.com/NCEA

National Council of Senior Citizens
8403 Colesville Rd., Suite 1200
Silver Spring, MD 20910-3314
1-888-3-SENIOR (1-800-373-6467)
Web site: www.ncscinc.org

National Institute on Aging Information Center (NIAIC)
P.O. Box 8057
Gaithersburg, MD 20898-8057
1-800-222-2225
TTY 1-800-222-4225
Web site: www.nih.gov/nia

AIDS/HIV

CDC National AIDS Hotline
P.O. Box 13827
RTP, NC 27709-3827
1-800-342-AIDS (1-800-342-2437)
(24 hours a day/7 days a week)
TTY 1-800-243-7889
Web site:
www.ashastd.org/nah/nah.html

HIV/AIDS Treatment Information Service
P.O. Box 6303
Rockville, MD 20849-6303
1-800-HIV-0440 (1-800-448-0440)
TTY 1-888-480-3739
E-mail: atis@hivatis.org
Web site: www.hivatis.org

Project Inform
205 13th St., #2001
San Francisco, CA 94103
1-800-822-7422 (Treatment Hotline phone number)
E-mail: web@ProjectInform.org
Web site: www.ProjectInform.org

ALTERNATIVE MEDICINE

National Center for Complementary and Alternative Medicine
P.O. Box 8218
Silver Spring, MD 20907-8218
1-888-644-6226
TTY 1-888-644-6226
Web site: http://nccam.nih.gov

ALZHEIMER'S DISEASE

Alzheimer's Association
919 N. Michigan Ave., Suite 1100
Chicago, IL 60611-1676
1-800-272-3900
Web site: www.alz.org

Alzheimer's Disease Education and Referral (ADEAR) Center
P.O. Box 8250
Silver Spring, MD 20907-8250
1-800-438-4380
E-mail: adear@alzheimers.org
Web site: www.alzheimers.org
A service of the National Institute on Aging (NIA)

ARTHRITIS

Arthritis Foundation
P.O. Box 7669
Atlanta, GA 30357-0669
1-800-283-7800
Web site: www.arthritis.org

National Institute of Arthritis and Musculoskeletal and Skin Diseases Information Clearinghouse
Office of Communications and Public Liaison
Building 31/Room 4C05
31 Center Dr., MSC 2350
Bethesda, MD 20892-2350
1-887-22-NIAMS (1-800-226-4267)
TTY 1-301-565-2966
Web site: www.nih.gov/niams

BONE HEALTH

American Academy of Orthopaedic Surgeons
6300 N. River Rd.
Rosemont, IL 60018-4262
1-800-346-AAOS (1-800-346-2267)
Web site: www.aaos.org

American Orthopaedic Foot and Ankle Society
1216 Pine St., Suite 201
Seattle, WA 98101
1-206-223-1120
E-mail: aofas@aofas.org
Web site: www.aofas.org

NIH Osteoporosis and Related Bone Diseases National Resource Center
1232 22nd St. NW
Washington, DC 20037-1292
1-800-624-BONE (1-800-624-2663)
TTY 1-202-466-4315
Web site: www.osteo.org

National Osteoporosis Foundation
1232 22nd St. NW
Washington, DC 20037-1292
1-800-223-9994 (24 hours a day/
7 days a week)
Web site: www.nof.org

CANCER

American Cancer Society
1599 Clifton Rd., NE
Atlanta, GA 30329-4251
1-800-227-2345
Web site: www.cancer.org

Cancer Care, Inc.
275 7th Ave.
New York, NY 10001
1-800-813-HOPE (1-800-813-4673)
E-mail: info@cancercare.org
Web site: www.cancercare.org
Cancer patient advocacy; Web site lists organizations that focus on specific diagnoses.

Cancer Liaison Program
Office of Special Health Issues
Food and Drug Administration
5600 Fishers Lane, HF-12, Room 9-49
Rockville, MD 20857
1-888-INFOFDA (1-800-463-6332)
E-mail: OSHI@oc.fda.gov
Web site: www.fda.gov/oashi/cancer/cancer.html
Provides information about the FDA drug approval process, cancer clinical trials, and access to investigational therapies.

National Alliance of Breast Cancer Organizations (NABCO)
9 E. 37th St., 10th floor
New York, NY 10016
1-888-806-2226
E-mail: NABCOinfo@aol.com
Web site: www.nabco.org

National Cancer Institute
Cancer Information Service
Building 31, 9000 Rockville Pike
Bethesda, MD 20892
1-800-4-CANCER (1-800-422-6237)
TTY 1-800-332-8615
Web site: www.nci.nih.gov

**National Coalition for Cancer
Survivorship**
1010 Wayne Ave., Suite 707
Silver Spring, MD 20910-5600
1-877-NCCS-YES (1-877-622-7937)
E-mail: info@cansearch.org
Web site: www.cansearch.org

DENTAL HEALTH

American Dental Association
211 E. Chicago Ave.
Chicago, IL 60611
1-800-947-4746
Web site: www.ada.org

DIABETES

American Diabetes Association
1701 North Beauregard St.
Alexandria, VA 22311
1-800-DIABETES (1-800-342-2383)
Web site: www.diabetes.org

**National Institute of Diabetes and
Digestive and Kidney Diseases (NIDDK)**
Office of Communications and
Public Liaison-NIDDK
31 Center Dr., MSC 2560
Bethesda, MD 20892-2560
1-800-891-5390
Web site: www.niddk.nih.gov

HEALTH AND WELL-BEING

**American College of Emergency
Physicians**
P.O. Box 619911
Dallas, TX 75261-9911
1-800-798-1822
Web site: www.acep.org

American Medical Association
515 North State St.
Chicago, IL 60610
1-312-464-5000
Web site: www.ama-assn.org
Online Doctor Finder: www.ama-
assn.org/aps/amahg.htm

Healthfinder
Web site: www.healthfinder.gov
This site is a gateway linking
consumers to health and human
services information from the federal
government and its many partners.

**Joint Commission on Accreditation
of Healthcare Organizations**
One Renaissance Blvd.
Oakbrook Terrace, IL 60181
1-630-792-5000
Web site: www.jcaho.org

National Women's Health Network
514 10th St. NW, Suite 400
Washington, DC 20004
1-202-628-7814
Web site:
www.womenshealthnetwork.org

**Office of Disease Prevention and
Health Promotion**
U. S. Department of Health and
Human Services
National Health Information Center
P. O. Box 1133
Washington, DC 20013-1133
Web site:
www.odphp.osophs.dhhs.gov

HEARING

International Hearing Society
16880 Middlebelt Rd., Suite 4
Livonia, MI 48154-3367
1-800-521-5247
Web site: www.hearingihs.org

Self Help for Hard of Hearing People, Inc.
7910 Woodmont Ave., Suite 1200
Bethesda, MD 20814
1-301-657-2248
TTY 1-301-657-2249
Web site: www.shhh.org

National Institute on Deafness and Other Communication Disorders
31 Center Dr., MSC 2320
Bethesda, MD 20892-2320
1-800-241-1044
TTY 1-800-241-1055
Web site: www.nih.gov/nidcd

HEART DISEASE

American Heart Association
7272 Greenville Ave.
Dallas, TX 75231
Customer Heart and Stroke
Information
1-800-AHA-USA1 (1-800-242-8721)
Stroke Information
1-888-4-STROKE (1-888-478-7653)
Women's Health Information
1-888-MY HEART (1-888-694-3278)
Web site: www.americanheart.org

LUNG DISEASE

American Lung Association
1740 Broadway
New York, NY 10019
1-800-LUNG-USA (1-800-586-4872)
E-mail: info@lungusa.org
Web site: www.lungusa.org

MENTAL HEALTH

American Psychiatric Association
1400 K St. NW
Washington, DC 20005
1-202-682-6000
E-mail: apa@psych.org
Web site: www.psych.org

National Alliance for the Mentally Ill
Colonial Place Three
2107 Wilson Blvd., Suite 300
Arlington, VA 22201-3042
1-800-950-NAMI (1-800-950-6264)
TDD 1-703-516-7227
Web site: www.nami.org

National Depressive and Manic-Depressive Association
730 N. Franklin St., Suite 501
Chicago, IL 60610-3526
1-800-82-NDMDA (1-800-826-3632)
1-888-425-4410 (for a depression
screening site in your area)
Web site: www.ndmda.org

National Foundation for Depressive Illness, Inc.
P.O. Box 2257
New York, NY 10116
1-800-239-1265
Web site: www.depression.org

National Institute of Mental Health
6001 Executive Blvd.,
Room 8184, MSC 9663
Bethesda, MD 20892-9663
1-800-64-PANIC (1-800-647-2642)
1-888-8-ANXIETY (1-888-826-9438)
Web site: www.nimh.nih.gov

National Mental Health Association
1021 Prince St.
Alexandria, VA 22314-2971
1-703-684-7722
1-800-969-NMHA (1-800-969-6642)
TTY 1-800-433-5959
Web site: www.nmha.org
Free screening test at
www.depression-screening. org

The THEOS International Foundation (THEOS)
322 Boulevard of the Allies, Suite 105
Pittsburgh, PA 15222-1919
1-412-471-7779
An international support network for recently widowed men and women.

NUTRITION

American Dietetic Association
216 W. Jackson Blvd.
Chicago, IL 60606
1-800-366-1655 (Nutrition
Information Hotline)
Web site: www.eatright.org

Food and Nutrition Information Center
Agricultural Research Service,
USDA National Agricultural Library,
Room 304
10301 Baltimore Ave.
Beltsville, MD 20705-2351
1-301-504-5755
TTY 1-301-504-6856
E-mail: fnic@nal.usda.gov
Web site: www.nal.usda.gov/fnic

PARKINSON'S DISEASE

American Parkinson's Disease Association
1250 Hylan Blvd., Suite 4B
Staten Island, NY 10305-1946
1-800-223-2732
Web site: www.apdaparkinson.com

National Parkinson Foundation, Inc.
Bob Hope Parkinson Research Center
1501 NW 9th Ave.
Miami, FL 33136-1494
1-800-327-4545
E-mail: mailbox@npf.med.miami.edu
Web site: www.parkinson.org

Parkinson's Disease Foundation
William Black Medical Building
Columbia-Presbyterian Medical
Center
710 West 168th St.
New York, NY 10032-9982
1-800-457-6676
E-mail: info@pdf.org
Web site: www.pdf.org

PATIENT/CAREGIVER ADVOCACY

**National Family Caregivers
Association**
10400 Connecticut Ave., #500
Kensington, MD 20895-3944
1-800-896-3650
E-mail: info@nfcacares.org
Web site: www.nfcacares.org

**National Hospice and Palliative Care
Organization**
(formerly known as the National
Hospice Organization)
1700 Diagonal Rd., Suite 300
Alexandria, VA 22314
1-800-658-8898
Web site: www.nhpco.org

Patient Advocate Foundation
753 Thimble Shoals Blvd., Suite B
Newport News, VA 23606
1-800-532-5274
E-mail: help@patientadvocate.org
Web site: www.patientadvocate.org
Serves as an active liaison between
patients and their insurers,
employers, and/or creditors.

SAFETY

**National Center for Injury
Prevention and Control**
Mailstop K65
4770 Buford Highway, NE
Atlanta, GA 30341-3724
1-770-488-1506
E-mail: OHCINFO@cdc.gov
Web site: www.cdc.gov/ncipc

National Safety Council
1121 Spring Lake Dr.
Itasca, IL 60143-3201
1-800-621-7619
Web site: www.nsc.org

SLEEP DISORDERS

**American Academy of Sleep
Medicine**
6301 Bandel Rd., NW, Suite 101
Rochester, MN 55901
1-507-287-6006
Web site: www.asda.org

American Sleep Apnea Association
1424 K St. NW, Suite 302
Washington, DC 20005
1-202-293-3650
E-mail: asaa@sleepapnea.org
Web site: www.sleepapnea.org

National Sleep Foundation
1522 K St. NW, Suite 500
Washington, DC 20005
1-202-347-3471
E-mail: nsf@sleepfoundation.org
Web site: www.sleepfoundation.org

STROKE

American Heart Association
7272 Greenville Ave.
Dallas, TX 75231
Stroke Information
1-888-4-STROKE (1-888-478-7653)
Web site: www.americanheart.org

National Institute of Neurological Disorders and Stroke
Office of Communications and
Public Liaison
P.O. Box 5801
Bethesda, MD 20824
1-800-352-9424
Web site: www.ninds.nih.gov

National Stroke Association
9707 East Easter Lane
Englewood, CO 80112-3747
1-800-STROKES (1-800-787-6537)
E-mail: info@stroke.org
Web site: www.stroke.org

SUBSTANCE ABUSE

Al-Anon Family Group Headquarters
1600 Corporate Landing Parkway
Virginia Beach, VA 23454
1-757-563-1600
1-888-4AL-ANON (1-888-425-2666)
(for meeting information)
E-mail: WSO@al-anon.org
Web site: www.al-anon.org

Alcoholics Anonymous World Services
P.O. Box 459, Grand Central Station
New York, NY 10163
1-212-870-3400
Web site: www.aa.org

Narcotics Anonymous World Service
P. O. Box 9999
Van Nuys, CA 91409
1-818-773-9999
E-mail: FSTeam@na.org
Web site: www.na.org

National Council on Alcoholism and Drug Dependence
12 West 21st St.
New York, NY 10010
1-212-206-6770
1-800-NCA-CALL (1-800-622-2255)
(24-hour affiliate referral)
Web site: www.ncadd.org

The National Clearinghouse for Alcohol and Drug Information (NCADI)
P.O. Box 2345
Rockville, MD 20847-2345
1-800-729-6686
TDD 1-800-487-4889
E-mail: info@health.org
Web site: www.health.org

National Institute on Drug Abuse
6001 Executive Blvd.
Bethesda, MD 20892-9561
1-301-443-1124
Web site: www.nida.nih.gov

UROLOGICAL DISORDERS

American Foundation for Urologic Disease
1128 North Charles St.
Baltimore, MD 21201
1-800-242-2383
Web site: www.incontinence.org

American Urological Association
1120 North Charles St.
Baltimore, MD 21201
1-410-727-1100
Web site: www.auanet.org
1-877-DRY-LIFE (1-877-379-5433)
(female incontinence info)
Web site: www.drylife.org

National Association for Continence
P.O. Box 8310
Spartanburg, SC 29305
1-800-BLADDER (1-800-252-3337)
Web site: www.nafc.org

National Institute of Diabetes and Digestive and Kidney Diseases (NIDDK)
Office of Communications and
Public Liaison-NIDDK
31 Center Dr., MSC 2560
Bethesda, MD 20892-2560
1-800-891-5390
Web site: www.niddk.nih.gov

National Kidney Foundation
30 East 33rd St., Suite 1100
New York, NY 10016
1-800-622-9010
Web site: www.kidney.org

The Prostatitis Foundation
1063 30th St., Box 8
Smithshire, IL 61478
1-888-891-4200
Web site: www.prostate.org

The Simon Foundation for Continence
P.O. Box 835-F
Wilmette, IL 60091
1-800-23-SIMON (1-800-237-4666)
Web site: www.simonfoundation.org

VISION

American Council of the Blind
1155 15th St. NW, Suite 1004
Washington, DC 20005
1-800-424-8666
Web site: www.acb.org

American Foundation for the Blind
11 Penn Plaza, Suite 300
New York, NY 10001
1-800-AFB-LINE (1-800-232-5463)
E-mail: afbinfo@afb.net
Web site: www.afb.org

Lighthouse International
111 East 59th St.
New York, NY 10022-1202
1-800-829-0500; 1-800-334-5497
TTY 1-212-821-9713
E-mail: info@lighthouse.org
Web site: www.lighthouse.org

National Association for the Visually Handicapped
22 W. 21st St., 6th floor
New York, NY 10010
1-212-889-3141
Web site: www.navh.org

National Eye Institute
2020 Vision Pl.
Bethesda, MD 20892-3655
1-301-496-5248
Web site: www.nei.nih.gov

OTHER RESOURCES

American Automobile Association
Web site: www.aaa.com

American Red Cross
431 18th St. NW
Washington, DC 20006
1-202-639-3520
E-mail: info@usa.redcross.org
Web site: www.redcross.org

Council of Better Business Bureaus, Inc.
4200 Wilson Blvd., Suite 800
Arlington, VA 22203-1838
1-703-276-0100
Web site: www.bbb.org

Corporation for National Service: Senior Corps
1201 New York Ave. NW
Washington, DC 20525
1-202-606-5000
E-mail: webmaster@cns.gov
Web site: www.seniorcorps.org

Environmental Protection Agency
Indoor Air Quality Publications, Radon-Specific
National Center for Environmental Publications
P.O. Box 42419
Cincinnati, OH 42419
1-800-490-9198
Web site: www.epa.gov/iaq/radon/pubs/index.html

Indian Health Service (IHS)
Room 6-35, Parklawn Building
5600 Fishers Lane
Rockville, MD 20857
1-301-443-3593
Web site: www.ihs.gov

TRICARE/Military DoD Health Affairs
Skyline 5, Suite 810
5111 Leesburg Pike
Falls Church, VA 22041-3206
Web site: www.tricare.osd.mil

United Way of America
701 N. Fairfax St.
Alexandria, VA 22314-2045
1-703-836-7100
Web site: www.unitedway.org

Veterans Health Administration (VHA)
1-800-827-1000
Web site: www.va.gov/vbs/health
The VHA provides a broad spectrum of medical, surgical, and rehabilitative care to veterans.

Personal Health History

(Use this form to make as many copies as you and your family need.)

Name: _____

Date of Birth: _____ Blood Type: _____

History of Childhood Diseases

Disease	Date of Illness	Disease	Date of Illness
Chicken Pox	_____	Measles	_____
Ear infection	_____	Mononucleosis	_____
German measles (rubella)	_____	Mumps	_____
		Polio	_____
Hepatitis	_____	Scarlet fever	_____

History of Chronic Diseases

(may include anemia or other blood disorder, arthritis, asthma, cancer, cataracts, diabetes, epilepsy, gastrointestinal disorder, glaucoma, heart disease, high cholesterol level, high blood pressure, kidney disease, mental illness, sexually transmitted diseases, or ulcer)

Disease: _____ Date Diagnosed: _____

Treatment: _____

_____

_____

Disease: _____ Date Diagnosed: _____

Treatment: _____

_____

_____

Disease: _____ Date Diagnosed: _____

Treatment: _____

_____

_____

Diseasc: _____ Date Diagnosed: _____

Treatment: _____

_____

_____

Family Health History

(Use this form to make as many copies as you and your family need.)

Knowing your family's health history is important to your own health. Record all known health conditions of your immediate relatives. Include your grandparents, parents, siblings, aunts, and uncles. While you should note conditions such as heart disease, high blood pressure, epilepsy, and liver disease, be sure to also include conditions such as cataracts, glaucoma, allergies, asthma, and ulcers. The more complete your history is, the better your doctor can assess your health risks.

Mother: _____

Conditions: _____

Cause of Death: _____ Age at Death: _____

Father: _____

Conditions: _____

Cause of Death: _____ Age at Death: _____

Grandparent: _____

Conditions: _____

Cause of Death: _____ Age at Death: _____

Grandparent: _____

Conditions: _____

Cause of Death: _____ Age at Death: _____

Other Relation: _____

Conditions: _____

Cause of Death: _____ Age at Death: _____

Other Relation: _____

Conditions: _____

Cause of Death: _____ Age at Death: _____

Other Relation: _____

Conditions: _____

Cause of Death: _____ Age at Death: _____

Screenings and Immunizations

(Use this form to make as many copies as you and your family need.)

Regular screenings are vital to your continued good health. Ask your doctor about which screenings, such as those that check cholesterol, blood pressure, cancer, and osteoporosis, are appropriate for you, and how often you should have them.

Regular Screenings	Date	Results	Next Due

Immunizations can help keep you going strong. Follow your doctor's recommendations regarding annual flu shots and immunizations against pneumonia, tetanus, diphtheria, and other preventable illnesses.

Immunizations	Date	Results	Next Due

Healthful lifestyle actions recommended by your doctor: _____ _____

_____

_____

Medication Record

(Use this form to make as many copies as you and your family need.)

Record all medicines you take—including prescription and over-the-counter drugs. Remember that vitamins and supplements, including herbal remedies, can affect the medicines you take, so be sure to include those as well. Tape this chart to the inside of your medicine cabinet. Take it with you when you visit your doctor.

Drug or Supplement: _____
Purpose: _____
Dose: _____
Instructions: _____
Date started: _____

Drug or Supplement: _____
Purpose: _____
Dose: _____
Instructions: _____
Date started: _____

Drug or Supplement: _____
Purpose: _____
Dose: _____
Instructions: _____
Date started: _____

Drug or Supplement: _____
Purpose: _____
Dose: _____
Instructions: _____
Date started: _____

Drug or Supplement: _____
Purpose: _____
Dose: _____
Instructions: _____
Date started: _____

Drug or Supplement: _____
Purpose: _____
Dose: _____
Instructions: _____
Date started: _____

Drug or Supplement: _____
Purpose: _____
Dose: _____
Instructions: _____
Date started: _____

Drug or Supplement: _____
Purpose: _____
Dose: _____
Instructions: _____
Date started: _____

Index

Index